D0059910

DISCARD

"More topical cases from Dr. Henry Lee to educate and entertain: from the headlines to the reader. Insightful commentary on cases in the news with perspectives only Dr. Lee can provide."

—Haskell M. Pitluck, retired Illinois circuit court judge and past president of the American Academy of Forensic Sciences

"Drs. Lee and Labriola have, once again, produced an excellent compilation of cases that have served to make Henry Lee a household name around the world. Having led the FBI's forensic science effort in mass grave excavations in Kosovo, I was moved by the exceptional chapter on the atrocities in Bosnia and Croatia for its historical background, the significant role played by forensic science in cases of war crimes, and Dr. Lee's unshakable optimism and self-deprecating humor."

—Dwight E. Adams, PhD, director, Forensic Science Institute, University of Central Oklahoma, and former director, FBI Laboratory

MORE ADVANCE PRAISE FOR *SHOCKING CASES*

"Dr. Henry C. Lee is the twenty-first century's version of Sherlock Holmes. His powers of observation are equaled only by his desire to share his expertise with law enforcement throughout the world. *Shocking Cases* demonstrates Dr. Lee's keen investigative talents and is a must read for all professional and amateur detectives."

—Mike Bottoms, district attorney general,
22nd Judicial District of Tennessee, and president of SELETS
(Southeastern Law Enforcement Training Seminars)

"Dr. Lee's world-renowned expertise in the field of forensic science has made him an insider to some of the most infamous cases of the century. From the JFK assassination to the O. J. Simpson murder case to JonBenet Ramsey, Dr. Lee has been brought in to explain what happened based on the science. In this book he once again examines headline-making cases from Phil Spector to Bosnian war crimes. This book gives an insider's look at these crimes. As Dr. Lee says, 'Science does not lie.'"

—Paul Connick Jr., district attorney, Jefferson Parish, Louisiana

"Frankly I am not sure which is more shocking, the abhorrent manner in which humans can treat one another or the sad reality that many horrific crimes go unsolved until the full potential of modern-day forensic science is integrated into the investigative plan. Once again, thank you Dr. Lee for helping resolve some of these complex crimes and sharing what you have learned so that we too may provide a solution to future crimes and provide some sense of peace to those who have been left behind in the wake of violence."

—Professor Timothy Palmbach, Forensic Science Department,
University of New Haven

SHOCKING CASES

SHOCKING CASES

FROM
DR. HENRY LEE'S
FORENSIC FILES

THE PHIL SPECTOR CASE
THE PRIEST'S RITUAL MURDER OF A NUN
THE BROWN'S CHICKEN MASSACRE AND MORE!

DR. HENRY C. LEE
AND
JERRY LABRIOLA, MD

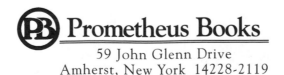

Prometheus Books

59 John Glenn Drive
Amherst, New York 14228-2119

Published 2010 by Prometheus Books

Inquiries should be addressed to
Prometheus Books
59 John Glenn Drive
Amherst, New York 14228–2119
VOICE: 716–691–0133
FAX: 716–691–0137
WWW.PROMETHEUSBOOKS.COM

14 13 12 11 10   5 4 3 2 1

Library of Congress Cataloging-in-Publication Data

Lee, Henry C.
    Shocking cases from Dr. Henry Lee's forensic files / by Henry C. Lee and Jerry Labriola.
        p. cm.
    Includes bibliographical references and index.
    ISBN 978–1–59102–775–1 (cloth : alk. paper)
    1. Criminal investigation—United States. 2. Case studies, Evidence, Criminal—United States. 3. Cases, Evidence, Criminal—Europe, Eastern. 4. Case studies. I. Title.

HV8073.L395 2010
363.25/95230973—dc22

2009039257

All photographs courtesy of Dr. Henry C. Lee
Printed in the United States of America

To our wives and children
To those members of law enforcement
and the scientific community
who worked diligently on these cases

CONTENTS

PROLOGUE

This is the fourth book we have coauthored. In its first four chapters, we examine the forensic evidence of major criminal cases taken from Dr. Lee's personal files. The fifth and final chapter deals with his experiences during the investigation of certain atrocities in southeastern Europe.

The geographic settings for the first four chapters stretch across the United States—Los Angeles, California; Chicago, Illinois; Toledo, Ohio; and Hartford, Connecticut—and the last one takes us to Bosnia and Croatia.

While our primary focus is forensic in nature, the cases discussed here involve such disparate subjects as Hollywood's music industry, Prohibition and organized crime, murder within a religious enclave, the dangers inherent in law enforcement and racial tension, and so-called ethnic cleansing.

As in our previous collaborations, brief expanded discussions are scattered throughout most chapters in this book. They are designated as sidebars and relate to the specific topic at hand.

Finally, any reference to "I," "me," or "my" refers to Dr. Lee.

Henry Lee, PhD
Jerry Labriola, MD

1

THE PHIL SPECTOR CASE

W e begin with a criminal case that rocked the suburbs of Los Angeles and beyond.

BACKGROUND

Phil Spector has been variously described as temperamental, brilliant, quirky—and sometimes violent. He has nonetheless made a mark as one of the giants in the music industry, more so as a record producer and songwriter than a performer. As we shall see, his life has been both glamorous and sordid, with stretches of enormous success and unexpected failure—or all of the above in the same month. Once called a "little man with lifts in his shoes, [with a] wig on top of his head and four guns,"[1] he's had tales of flaunting of firearms—including confronting performers with a gun or laughing while pointing a loaded pistol at a fellow producer's head—haunt him. Such gunplay took a different turn, however, in 2003, when he was arrested on suspicion of the murder of an attractive forty-year-old actress named Lana Clarkson.

The Early Years

Harvey Philip Spector was born December 26, 1939, in the Bronx, where he learned to play guitar and piano at an early age. Even then he had visions of becoming a songwriter, session musician, and record producer. Following his father's death by suicide in 1949, he moved with his family to Los Angeles, and it was there that he immersed himself in all aspects of the music business. He and three high school friends formed a band called the Teddy Bears. They (and especially Spector as both songwriter and performer) burst onto the musical scene with songs that impressed several record companies. One ballad—"To Know Him Is to Love Him"—went to number one on *Billboard*'s Hot 100 singles chart in 1958, selling more than a million copies in a matter of months. He was a seventeen-year-old high school student at the time and had taken the title from the inscription on his father's gravestone. At such a young age, Spector was well on his way to becoming a millionaire. Although the group dissolved soon thereafter, nearly thirty years later the song became a hit again when Dolly Parton, Emmylou Harris, and Linda Ronstadt, working as a trio, reprised it in 1987.

From 1958 to 1966, Spector concentrated mainly on production, forming a new record company, cooperating with others, and working freelance with established artists. But he didn't abandon songwriting entirely; during this time he penned such hits as "On Broadway" for the Drifters, "Spanish Harlem" for Ben E. King, and "You've Lost That Lovin' Feelin'" for the Righteous Brothers. The latter is cited by Broadcast Music Incorporated (BMI) as the song with the most US airtime in the twentieth century. There were flops during this period, to be sure, but he seemed to take them in stride, immediately bouncing back with a vengeance—and another smash hit.

As a producer, he turned out blockbusters such as "Zip-a-Dee-Doo-Dah," "My Sweet Lord," "River Deep—Mountain High," "Just Once in My Life," "Unchained Melody," "Ebb Tide," and "Every Breath I Take." Also among his productions was the Beatles' colossal album *Let It Be*, and between 1960 and 1965, he produced more than twenty-five top 40 hits.

Spector's innovative trademark during the sixties was the dramatic Wall of Sound, a production technique that utilized large numbers of musicians to create a dense and thunderous effect. The process combined scores of instruments, sound effects, and vocals—overdubbing in duplicate or triplicate to create the layered, textured quality that he wanted. Spector himself called his technique "a Wagnerian approach to rock and roll: little symphonies for the kids."[2] Sometimes enormous groups of musicians took part: two bassists, three guitarists, three pianists, two or three drummers, and other percussionists.

During this era he usually worked at the Los Angeles Gold Star Studios because of its echo chambers that were so essential to his Wall of Sound. This technique is what made him such an important figure in the music world. Microphones in the recording studio would capture the sound, which was then transmitted to an echo chamber outfitted with speakers and microphones. The signal from the studio, playing through the speakers, would reverberate around the room before being picked up by the microphones. The echo-laden sound was then channeled back to the control room, where it was transferred to tape. The natural reverberation and echo from the hard walls of the room gave his productions their distinctive sound, and when played on AM radio it resulted in a rich and complex quality with an impressive depth rarely heard in mono recordings. Songwriter Jeff Barry described the Wall of Sound as "basically a formula. You're going to have four or five guitars line up, gut-string guitars, and they're going to follow the chords...two basses in fifths, with the same type of line and strings...six or seven horns, adding the little punches...formula percussion instruments—the little bells, the shakers, the tambourines. Phil used his own formula for echo, and some overtone arrangements with strings. But by and large there was a formula arrangement."[3]

Spector's signature design changed the way pop records were created and brought fame to singing groups such as the Crystals and the Ronettes (whose lead singer, Ronnie Bennett, he married in 1968), among others.

It was almost inevitable that Spector would devise such a revolutionary new sound, because he had many unconventional ideas about musical and recording techniques. For example, he openly detested stereo releases, claiming they took control of the record's sound away from the producer and gave it to the listener. He was just as vocal in his opposition to albums, once characterizing them as "two hits and ten pieces of junk."[4]

He used an uncharacteristically hands-off approach, however, in working with his favorite musicians, a core collection of session players he affectionately labeled the "Wrecking Crew." Its members included guitarist Glen Campbell, pianist Leon Russell, and drummer Hal Blaine.

In 1971 Spector coproduced John Lennon's chart-topping *Imagine* album, utilizing forty-four microphones simultaneously. Its title track—which hit number one after Lennon's murder in 1980—is widely considered among the greatest pop songs of all time. But his relationship with Lennon soon soured. Some unnamed sources claimed Spector suffered a nervous breakdown in a recording studio and even brandished a gun in front of the famous Beatle. Also in 1971, Spector recorded the music for the number one triple album *The Concert for Bangladesh*, which captured the "Album of the Year" award at the 1972 Grammys.

The Later Years

Having created the unique Wall of Sound, producing hit after hit, and working successfully with artists such as the Beatles, Tina Turner, Connie Francis, Celine Dion, Cher, and the Ramones—all just a part of his legendary musical output—Spector was inducted into the Rock and Roll Hall of Fame as a nonperformer in 1989. And in 2004 *Rolling Stone* magazine ranked him sixty-third on its list of the 100 Greatest Artists of All Time.[5]

But in earlier decades—especially during the seventies—Spector began to exhibit erratic behavior and grew increasingly reclusive. His personality became more prickly. Friends labeled him controlling; those not so friendly stamped him as an outright paranoid. Even his appearance changed: Some called his attire "off the wall," while his signature mounds of curly hair seemed to turn wilder and more variegated. And he was noted for suddenly whipping out a handgun from his waistband and waving it menacingly before people.

"It had to stop," Spector said of his behavior in a 1977 *Los Angeles Times* interview. "Being the rich millionaire in the mansion and then dressing up as Batman. I have to admit I did enjoy it to a certain extent. But I began to realize it was very unhealthy."[6]

In the mid-1990s he allegedly ranted on about a singer's handlers and their lack of respect for his own legendary status. "You don't tell Shakespeare what plays to write," he groused, "or how to write them."[7] He later told a British writer that he was taking medication for schizophrenia. "But I wouldn't say I'm schizophrenic," he commented. "I [just] have devils inside that fight me."[8]

FACTS OF THE CASE

The Victim

On the morning of February 3, 2003, forty-year-old Lana Clarkson, a beautiful six-foot-tall actress, was found shot to death in the marble foyer of Spector's hilltop mansion in Alhambra, a suburb of Los Angeles. Police were summoned to the gated estate on Grandview Drive at around 5:00 a.m. by Spector's limousine driver. The driver, Adriano DeSouza, had called 911 on his cell phone to report hearing a gunshot.

Clarkson was born in Southern California and raised in Cloverdale. Friends said she'd been inspired by Marilyn Monroe, but she never quite fulfilled her early A-list dreams. She had to settle as a cult figure in B-movies and eventually sold her pinups on the Internet as her career faded.

Among her films were *The Haunting of Morella, Amazon Women on the Moon,* and *Barbarian Queen,* which she called the template for the hit TV series *Xena: Warrior Princess.* She also had small roles in *Scarface* and *Fast Times at Ridgemont High,* and made many appearances in commercials for companies like Kmart and television shows from *Silk Stalkings* and *Black Scorpion* on cable to NBC's *Knight Rider.*

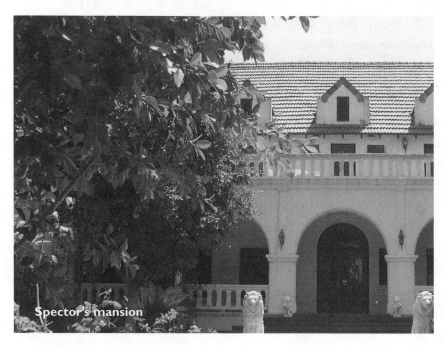

Spector's mansion

At age forty, stuck in a rut of low-budget, occasionally topless roles, she was struggling to make a living—yet she was said to be cheerful and smiling through it all. A month before her death, she began working at the House of Blues nightclub in West Hollywood's Sunset Strip, where she was a ticket collector and hostess. She rationalized to anyone who would listen that the move was an excellent opportunity to meet the "right" people, to work her way up in the film industry. That was her secret ambition, she would whisper in her best Monroe imitation.

"She wasn't thrilled to have people from the industry see her doing that, but she thought it was a good step to get back into the mainstream," said neighbor Paul Pietrewicz.[9]

Clarkson was also trying to jump-start her career by taking on theater parts. She did stand-up at the Comedy Club. She put together a Tracey Ullman–like tape of herself doing various comedic characters, among them Little Richard. And she networked relentlessly. "Everybody always knew Lana was in the room," ex-boyfriend Robert Hall said. "She was amazingly spunky, fun, energetic. By Hollywood standards, she was past her prime, but she worked it 100%—gave it more than you see most people giving it.... For as hard as she worked, I think she deserved recognition."[10]

Her small cult following continued to greet her at conventions and at events to publicize the TV shows she worked on. "She'd put in more hours, she'd stay more days," said actress Athena Massey, who met Clarkson when they worked together in *Black Scorpion*. "She was always trying to see how she could... find the next job or turn the job into something bigger."[11]

Most of those who mourned her passing referred to Clarkson as an indomitable woman, yet one who was increasingly aware of the challenges older actresses face. "Anyone over 40 is fighting uphill in this town," said friend and veteran actress Sally Kirkland. "But she was such a pro. She would come earlier than anybody, she would work harder than anybody."[12]

POLICE RESPONSE AND CRIMINAL INVESTIGATION

The following official report provides an indication of early police activity and investigative procedures in this case. In the interest of clarity, we have edited and/or slightly modified selected portions of the material, but in so doing, the accuracy of the information has not been compromised. The names of police officers and other investigators have been deleted.

ALHAMBRA POLICE DEPARTMENT
CRIME REPORT NARRATIVE
Date: 02/03/2003
S-Spector (Code: "S" refers to "Suspect") was placed under arrest... and transported to APD Jail for booking.... After S-Spector was transported, I [i.e., the police officer] went back up to the front doors of the house and was told by [a police corporal] that I was going to be the [evidence-]handling officer. I then advised [an officer] to start a major incident log.

I then interviewed R-Souza (Code: "R" refers to "Reporting Party") [actually, the correct spelling of the name is "DeSouza"] in front of the residence on Grandview. R-Souza stated that he is S-Spector's chauffeur and started work on 02/02/03 at 1900 hours. R-Souza stated that he drove S-Spector to several different locations over the night. At approx. 0200 hours on 02/03/03, R-Souza picked up S-Spector and a female who identified herself as "Lana" (Victim) at the House of Blues night club in Hollywood. R-Souza stated that he had never seen the female before.

At approx. 0300 hours, R-Souza pulled into the front of 1700 S. Grandview and S-Spector asked to be let out of the car at the bottom of the front stairway. S-Spector and the unidentified victim got out of the vehicle and proceeded up the stairway to the residence. R-Souza drove the vehicle around the back and parked it near the fountain. R-Souza then stated that it is routine for him to give S-Spector his luggage approx. 20 minutes after they arrive at his house. At approx. 0320 hours, R-Souza gave S-Spector his leather bag that contains his DVD player, cell phone, and other misc. personal items at the back door of the residence. R-Souza then returned to the car and sat in the vehicle for approx. two hours. At approx. 0455 hours, R-Souza heard a loud "Boom," and got out of the car. R-Souza stood by the vehicle for approx. five minutes and then closed the door to the car.

At this time, S-Spector opened the rear door to the residence. S-Spector was holding a black handgun in his right hand and stated, "I think I killed somebody." R-Souza stated that he saw blood on S-Spector's hands, but was not completely sure. R-Souza then saw the legs of the victim behind S-Spector, but could not see the rest of the body. R-Souza then moved a little to the side to get a better view of the victim and he saw the upper half of her body sitting in a chair just inside the door. R-Souza saw that there was blood on the left side of the victim's face and ran back to the vehicle. R-Souza got on his cell phone and telephoned S-Spector's secretary. R-Souza left a message on her machine stating that he thought that S-Spector shot someone. R-Souza drove down the driveway and out the front gates and dialed "911" on his cell phone. R-Souza waited out front for the police to arrive.

I spoke to [a police officer] who told me the following: [Several officers] received a [radio call] to respond to 1700 S. Grandview for a possible gun shot heard. Dispatch further advised that the caller's boss had a gun in his hand and a woman was shot inside the residence. [Two officers] responded to the backside of the residence off of Alta Vista and watched the back. The other officers set up a command post at the front of the residence off of Grandview. R-Souza gave them further information, including a suspect description.

[Several other officers] entered the property to investigate the call. While they were searching the garage to the rear of the residence, [one officer] observed a subject matching the description of the suspect on the stairway inside the residence. The subject (S-Spector) then walked out the open rear door and stood on the rear stairs with his hands in his front pants pockets. An [officer] repeatedly ordered S-Spector to raise his hands. S-Spector finally raised his hands quickly and then placed them back in his front pants pockets. S-Spector turned around and walked back into his house. The officers quickly approached the door, so that they would not lose sight of the suspect, at which time S-Spector turned around. They ordered him again to take his hands out of his front pants pockets, but he refused to remove them.

[An officer] then shot the air-taser at S-Spector, but one of the prongs did not stick. Since the taser was ineffective, [three officers] rushed S-Spector and knocked him to the ground. S-Spector was then handcuffed and detained at his residence. [An officer] observed a female sitting in the chair next to where they detained S-Spector. [The officer] checked the female for pulse, but found no signs of any pulse.[13]

When questioned later, the chauffeur stated he had transported Spector and a tall, beautiful woman he believed was named Lana to Spector's home, allegedly to have a drink. He added that the woman's car was a black Mercury Cougar that she had parked quite a distance from the House of Blues on Sunset Boulevard before they drove—in Spector's Mercedes-Benz—to his home on South Grandview. There, after leaving the couple off near the front entrance and driving to the rear of the home, he sat in the car for about two hours. It was then that he heard a shot ring out. The sound came from inside the house. Minutes later, he said, Spector appeared at the door holding a black handgun; DeSouza said he looked drunk.

"What happened, Sir?" the driver asked.

"I think I killed somebody," Spector reportedly responded.

Meanwhile, homicide detectives searched Spector's car and found nothing suspicious, and several again checked the body for a pulse and again found none. They noted that blood had drained from her ears, mouth, and nose; that her skin was cool to the touch; and that she showed no signs of life.

Conspicuous at the death scene was a small-caliber revolver with a brown wooden handle. It lay on the floor near the decedent's left calf. Also to her left was a desk with an open drawer. Inside, officers found a tan suede holster for a small-caliber weapon, presumably the one on the floor.

One of the officers claimed that the decedent appeared to have been placed in the chair after she sustained her injuries and that there were no signs that the shooting had occurred in the area where she was discovered.

Paramedics pronounced Clarkson dead at 6:25 a.m., and at about the same time, Spector was taken to the Alhambra Police Department and booked for suspicion of murder. The weapon, identified as a Colt Cobra .38 caliber revolver, was booked into evidence.

The day after the shooting, Spector's attorney, Robert Shapiro, asked forensic pathologist Dr. Michael Baden and me to examine Spector and the scene of the shooting. Our findings, along with my personal observations, are detailed later in this chapter. (See page 33.) For now, suffice it to say that the following particulars surfaced during the initial phase of the investigation. They pertain primarily to the examination of the body and to a description of the death scene.

The female victim—approximately forty years old—was found sitting stiffly in a chair, her legs extended straight out in front, her toes pointed inward. She was dressed in a black jacket top, a black lace and rhinestone decorated slip, black panties, black bra, black pantyhose, and black Mary Jane shoes. Her arms were down at her sides and over the arms of the chair. Her head was tilted to the left and flexed down slightly on her chest. Her upper central incisor teeth appeared to be broken and missing. A small bluish discolored area was noted below her left eye. A handbag was over her right shoulder and hung down over the side of the chair, reaching the floor. A moderate amount of blood was noted on the bag. Her face was bloodied about her nose and right cheek, and blood was draining from her right ear. Rigor mortis was present to the extent of 2+ in the neck, 3+ in the hips, and 4+ in the remainder of the body. These determinations were made at 7:18 p.m. Livor mortis was present and consistent with the body position. At 10:15 p.m., it was light to dark purple and did not blanch upon firm pressure. ("Rigor mortis" refers to the stiffening of the body after death due to postmortem muscle contraction. "Livor mortis"—also called "postmortem lividity"—is a reddish, purplish-blue discoloration of the skin due to settling of blood, by gravity, in the vessels of the dependent areas of the body. The higher the number, the greater the intensity.)

With regard to the scene, it was the rear ground-level foyer of Spector's residence. On the east side of the foyer was a sideboard with chairs on either side of it. Directly opposite, on the west side, was a staircase leading to the second floor. Clarkson's body was located in the northernmost chair. Just to her left and beneath her leg was a .38 caliber Colt Cobra. It was found to have five live rounds and one expended round of ammunition. Blood was noted on the weapon's grip and trigger guard, and the right side of its cylinder. Two taser darts and cords were seen on the carpeting in front of and to both sides of the body, while toward its front and near the staircase were two small white objects that appeared to be tooth material. Two additional fragments—apparently of the same material—were found halfway up the stairs. Several small blood spots were noted on the carpeting under the right side of the chair, next to Lana's handbag and right hand. Upon examination of the bag's contents, examiners discovered a black skirt and a pair of black dress gloves.

It should be mentioned that Lana's mother, Donna Clarkson, told police that her daughter had recently had new caps placed on her upper central incisors.

One aspect of the investigation that would receive considerable attention later at the trial had to do with the collection of gunshot residue from Lana's hands and tongue. So-called adhesive lift samples that contained such residue were obtained from both hands and from the upper surface of Lana's tongue. The conclusions drawn by the coroner's office were that (1) she may have discharged a firearm or had her hands otherwise in an environment of gunshot residue and (2) the upper surface of her tongue may have been in an environment of gunshot residue or received gunshot particles from an environmental source. (See the sidebar "Gunshot Residue and Scanning Electron Microscopy" below.)

In addition, forensic scientists examined the decedent under ultraviolet light and detected a small amount of fibrous material on the lower portion of her slip. Other significant findings were a small piece of white material on her dress/slip; a piece of coarse dark hair between her breasts; a lipstick container inside her bra; dark, bloodlike stains trailing down the right side of her jacket, onto the white chair, and finally onto the leopard-print handbag; and bloodlike stains on her dress/slip and on her hands and wrists. She was also found to have a chipped/broken right thumbnail. This would also receive much attention at the subsequent trial—some would claim *inordinate* attention.

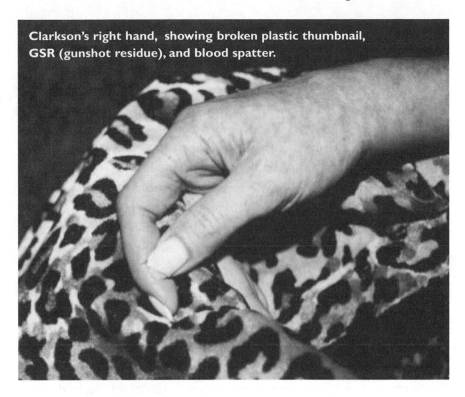

Clarkson's right hand, showing broken plastic thumbnail, GSR (gunshot residue), and blood spatter.

The autopsy report revealed the cause of death to be a gunshot wound of the head and neck, with entry being the oral cavity (mouth). The direction of the fatal bullet was front to back and slightly upward. Its course was described as oral cavity, the top portion of the tongue, the hard and soft palate, the back of the throat, the upper two cervical (neck) vertebrae, the upper spinal cord, and the occipital bone (base of the skull). There was no exit wound, and a projectile was found embedded in the occipital bone. It was a deformed copper jacket lead bullet.

Among the numerous injuries associated with the shooting, the major ones were fractures of facial bones, hard palate, upper two cervical vertebrae, and skull bones; lacerations of the tongue, soft palate, upper esophagus (gullet), back wall of the throat, the cervical spinal cord (complete); and various hemorrhages within the brain.

The autopsy report by Deputy Medical Examiner Louis A. Pena, MD, contained the following information:

> This 40-year-old Caucasian woman died as a result of a gunshot wound of the head and neck while in the accompaniment of a male at his residence. She was found slouched in a chair with her legs stretched out in front of her.
>
> Pertinent autopsy findings show a complete transection [cutting across] of the upper cervical spinal cord with associated fractures of the cervical vertebrae. The transection of the upper cervical spinal cord would result in immediate impairment with loss of respiratory and cardiac functions. In addition, there are basal skull fractures and associated intracerebral and brain-stem hemorrhages.
>
> The entrance wound of the oral cavity to include the tongue shows gunshot residue consistent with close range of fire. The Los Angeles County Sheriff's Department physical evidence examination supports the opinion that the weapon was in the mouth.
>
> Statements made in the law enforcement reports indicate that the male companion had possession of the gun when it was discharged. Circumstances also indicate that the weapon was apparently taken from a holster found in the drawer in the male companion's house left of the decedent's position.
>
> It should be noted that there was no history of suicidal ideations of the decedent and there was no suicide note found at the scene.

Based on the history, circumstances, law enforcement police reports, and autopsy, as currently known, the manner of death is homicide.[14]

Gunshot Residue and Scanning Electron Microscopy

When a firearm is discharged, gases, soot, and partially burned or unburned gunpowder, resulting from the detonation of the primer and the burning of gunpowder, are created. These materials are propelled forward with the projectile toward the target; at the same time, some of these materials are blown backward onto the shooter. These materials constitute the major components of gunshot residue (GSR). If samples are collected from the hands or clothing of the shooter prior to washing or removal by other means, GSR may be detected on these samples. The detection of GSR may aid in the identification of a shooter or the reconstruction of a shooting incident.

Among other materials, gunshot residue contains lead, barium, and antimony. (See below.) Modern forensic methods require the presence of these particles to identify trace evidence as GSR residue. Through the 1990s the presence of two or more of these elements was sufficient to conclude the chemicals were the result of a gunshot, but now more vigorous standards for GSR testing are being required by many courts.

GSR can originate from the primer, propellant, lubricant, and metals from the ammunition and barrel of a weapon.

Two common methods for the collection of GSR are SEM adhesive discs and AA swabs. It is important to note that gunshot residue may be removed from the hands by any activity, especially washing and cleaning. Thus, collection of such evidence should be conducted as soon as possible and always before fingerprinting.

Currently, the adhesive disc method is the preferred one. It utilizes scanning electron microscopy (SEM) for analysis. Commercially available kits contain either two or four discs per kit. Each hand and palm is patted with the adhesive disc to collect particles of GSR. Each should be patted until the adhesive properties of the disc are lost. At this point no further sampling should be conducted with that disc. The disc collection technique must be done before any other sampling technique in order to preserve the gunshot residue particle. Disposable gloves should be worn during the collection.

In the swab method, analysis is performed using an atomic absorption spectrometer (AA). Commercially available kits contain six or seven test tubes with swabs.

Gunshot residue analysis may be performed on other items of evidence such as clothing or vehicles.

The microscope is essential in the laboratory analysis of GSR. Examination for the presence of gunpowder particles, smudges, and burns around a bullet hole or in swabs from the hands is aided by the use of low-power magnification.

There are also chemical tests that may be used to show the distribution of residue on clothing and a target surface or as screening devices to locate areas that might be tested further. Commonly occurring substances such as cigarette smoke, urine, and fertilizer also react with some of these reagents. (Reagents are substances that, because of the reactions they cause, are used in chemical analysis.)

The methods employed in forensic laboratories for detecting the components of GSR are scanning electron microscopy, neutron activation analysis (NAA), gas chromatography/mass spectrometer (GC/MS), and high-performance liquid chromatography (HPLC). Only scanning electron microscopy will be discussed here (see below).

It should be pointed out that primer residues may help in another fashion. They adhere to fired bullets and gradually dissipate through the path of the bullet. Thus primer residue may be found on targets or in wound tracks at considerable distances from the gun muzzle.

Scanning Electron Microscopy (SEM) involves a microscope that uses electrons rather than light to form an image. Developed in the early 1950s, it has become a valuable instrument for study within the medical and physical sciences because it allows examination of a vast variety of specimens, including gunshot residue. The major benefits of the SEM image are its high magnification, high resolution, and great depth of focus. An optical microscope uses lenses to bend light waves, and the lenses are adjusted for focus. In the SEM, however, electromagnets bend an electron beam that is used to produce an image on a screen.

Gunshot residue particles can be identified by SEM according to their morphology (shape and structure). These particles are further studied by X-ray analysis for their elemental composition. A particle containing the elements of lead, barium, and antimony with a distinct morphology confirms the presence of gunshot residue.

GSR pattern analysis is valuable in the reconstruction of shooting events, especially in distance estimation. Interpretations are dependent upon the weapon used, the type of ammunition, the amount of load, whether or not an intermediate target was involved, and other factors. In general, GSR patterns on the target surface will have the following characteristics:

- **Contact shot** (end of gun is pressed against the skin). Soot deposits around the entrance hole. Very little or no unburned powder will be found.
- **Close-range shot**. Residues are deposited around the bullet hole with black soot and smoke. GSR particles can be found within a pattern that is small and dense.
- **Medium-range shot** (1.5 to 3 feet). Scattered gunshot residue is present without black soot deposits. The GSR pattern spreads out as the distance increases.
- **Long-range shot**. Gunpowder residue is usually not found on the target when the barrel to target dis-

tance is greater than five feet, although this may not be the case in instances where primer residue sticks to the fired bullet (as mentioned above).

Finally, one must not lose sight of the fact that the cartridge case, bullet, bullet coating, and metal jacket also contain specific elements that can be identified. Nearly all cartridge cases are made of brass (70 percent copper and 30 percent zinc). Bullet cores are most often lead and antimony, with a few having a ferrous alloy core. Bullet jackets are usually brass (90 percent copper and 10 percent zinc), but some are a ferrous alloy and some are aluminum.

In the physical examination of a crime scene or a body for evidence of gunshot residue, it must be remembered that glass particles contain lead, and these may mimic gunshot residue. Glass residue may be found up to thirty feet from the muzzle and are always present on the opposite side of a penetrated target. Such a situation may occur when a glass surface is present as an intermediate target.

From the beginning, the death of a fading actress in the home of a reclusive music mogul puzzled both police and friends alike. Stories quickly circulated that Spector and Clarkson were drunk, engaged in playful activity, and in the process, she was accidentally shot. Another story was that Clarkson, already depressed, rejected Spector's sexual advances and instead kissed the gun and took her own life. Still another was that it was an obvious case of murder, given the reputation of Spector with respect to his personality and his fascination with guns. In any event, he was hauled away to the Alhambra jail, but was released about twelve hours later after posting $1 million bail. He was accompanied by his lawyer, Robert Shapiro, who had also been part of the O. J. Simpson defense team.

Meanwhile, a large team of investigators (107 in all!), led by sheriff's detectives, forensic scientists from the crime lab and coroner's office, and crime scene technicians of the Los Angeles Sheriff's Department pored over Spector's wooded estate during the twenty-four hours after the killing. They paid special attention to the back foyer and the driveway where Spector's newly purchased Mercedes was parked facing the front gate, its driver's-side door still agape. They learned that he had purchased the thirty-three-room Alhambra château—built in 1926 and dubbed the Pyrenees Castle—for $1.1 million in 1998. In an interview for *Esquire* magazine shortly after the sale, Spector said he had bought "a beautiful and enchanting castle in a hick town where there is no place to go that you shouldn't go."[15]

Friends thought the new residence had somehow helped in rehabilitating the once-reckless producer, so they were generally flabbergasted by the charge levied against him. They were particularly perplexed about motive. "None of this equates," said guitarist Dave Kessel, one of Spector's closest friends. "He has been in great spirits and great shape, and feeling so good about everything. This doesn't fit into what I know about him and where he is."[16]

Eventually it was established that Spector began a busy evening on February 2—the night before Clarkson died—at the Beverly Hills restaurant The Grill on the Alley with a friend, Rommie Davis. In fact, they had dined together on three successive nights leading up to Clarkson's death. Later at the trial, Davis would testify that the producer had never in the past touched alcohol in her presence but now was suddenly ordering drinks, including two daiquiris at The Grill. She would say that he brushed her off when she warned that mixing alcohol with his medications could prove a lethal combination.

After his chauffeur drove Davis home, Spector returned to The Grill to pick up waitress Kathy Sullivan. They went to Trader Vic's—a Polynesian-themed restaurant in the Beverly Hilton—so Sullivan could eat dinner. While there, Spector ordered two Navy Grogs—a large cocktail with a frilly presentation. Prosecutors would later indicate that each of these drinks contains three shots of rum.

Next they drove to Dan Tana's, a celebrity hangout in West Holly-wood where Spector ordered two more daiquiris.

The last stop of the night—in the early morning hours of Feb-ruary 3—was the Foundation Room at the House of Blues nightclub, where Spector met Clarkson, apparently for the first time. There, he drank a shot of rum.

Both Davis and Sullivan would testify that he ordered food—prime ribs at The Grill and a salad at Dan Tana's—but only picked at the plates when they arrived.[17]

On February 4, the day after the killing, authorities searched Clarkson's Web site, where they learned of her admiration for Marilyn Monroe. "This is not to imply," she wrote in one posting, "that I wish to live the sort of lonely and narcotics-shrouded existence she did. What I love about her is her essence, her work and her commitment to it.... I have been blessed to work in an extremely difficult industry but in my opinion have not even begun to reach my full potential. I have been pounding my head against a Plexiglas ceiling trying to break through to a completely different level for a while now. God willing, this is the year it will happen. Keep your eye out for a new quality of work from Ms. Clarkson!"[18]

The attitude apparent in such a posting—as we have seen and will read more about later—did not jibe with those who believed Clarkson had taken her own life. Still, Spector sent e-mails to friends stating that he would be cleared and that her death would be ruled "an accidental suicide," a phrase some considered an oxymoron. And attorney Robert Shapiro told the Associated Press, "I am convinced that the thorough and accurate investigation of the evidence by the Los Angeles sheriff's department, its criminalists and the county coroner will prove that Phil Spector is innocent of any crime."[19]

But the rumor mill worked overtime. The press reported widely divergent assessments of Lana Clarkson: that she was very well liked, generous, and plucky; that she had once worked as a call girl—and worse.

As early as March, a sheriff's department statement said investiga-tors had discounted suicide as a possible cause of death, but Spector, in another *Esquire* interview, countered that Clarkson had "kissed the gun" before shooting herself. "I have no idea why," he said. "I never knew her, never even saw her before that night. I have no idea who she was or what her agenda was."

He went on to say he did not know where Clarkson got the gun that killed her, and that she was "loud and drunk" before leaving the House of Blues. "She asked me for a ride home. Then she wanted to see the castle," Spector said, referring to his suburban mansion. "She grabbed a bottle of tequila from the bar to take with her. I was not drunk. I wasn't drunk at all. There is no case. She killed herself.... It's 'Anatomy of a Frame-Up.' I didn't do anything wrong.... If they had a case, I'd be sitting in jail right now."[20]

He had not, in fact, been charged with a crime; authorities claimed they were still investigating the case. In June they announced publicly that it might take months to gather all the evidence and carry out complex forensic tests. Then, in September, sheriff's detectives proclaimed that Spector was responsible for the shooting death; they had submitted their findings to prosecutors. "It's not an accident. It's not a suicide," Captain Frank Merriman told the *Los Angeles Times*. "Phil Spector shot her." And the district attorney's office indicated that no immediate decision was expected on whether or not criminal charges would be filed.[21]

Two months later, the sixty-four-year-old Spector was formally charged with murder. Shapiro entered a plea of not guilty on his client's behalf, and Spector was allowed to remain free on $1 million bail, a decision that irked a hoard of detractors. At that time, sworn affidavits from witnesses and police were released about the night in question, providing different (and sometimes conflicting) details of what happened. In addition to elaborating on the body's location and position as well as the need for a Taser stun gun and brute force to corral Spector, official documents stated that officers found Clarkson's teeth scattered around the back foyer while a gun was found a few feet from her body. Also mentioned was that (1) authorities had characterized their meeting as a "sexual encounter" and (2) police had confiscated nine guns and a substantial quantity of ammunition from the residence.

THE PRETRIAL YEARS, 2003–2007

Much can happen during a prolonged pretrial period, and indeed that was the case here. Up to the mid-2007 trial, a virtual parade of defense lawyers—including Robert Shapiro, Marvin Mitchelson, Leslie Abramson, Marcia Morrissey, Bruce Cutler, Roger Rosen, and Bradley Brunon—represented the defendant, and each was eventually dismissed or resigned for one reason or another. Finally it was Linda Kenney-Baden, the wife of my good friend and forensic science colleague Dr. Michael Baden, who was retained by Spector and gave the defense's summation in September 2007.

Another incident occurred. Prosecutors alleged that the defense had withheld a mysterious piece of evidence from them. They claimed a torn piece of Clarkson's artificial fingernail had been overlooked by investigating officials. What's more, prosecutors stated that it was I who found the fingernail and that I had surreptitiously kept it. Such an absurd statement was then leaked to the news media, which then ran the story without checking its veracity. *The fact is that there never was a broken fingernail found at the scene.*

On February 4, 2003, Baden and I—having been contacted by Robert Shapiro—examined Spector for any scratches or other injuries that might have been the result of a struggle with Clarkson. We examined his body inch-by-inch and found none. At approximately 9:30 p.m., we went to Spector's house after the police had completed their investigation. We were accompanied by Shapiro, attorney Sara Caplan, and two private investigators—including Stanley White, with whom I would later have a major disagreement, as you will see. We were greeted by several Los Angeles detectives, and, upon the completion of their work there, they released the scene to us. We entered the back foyer, a relatively small area—no more than five by five feet. Clarkson's body, her purse, the gun, and most all other evidence had been collected and removed by Los Angeles Sheriff's Department officials. Among my personal notes were the following entries (note #9):

Location: 1st floor (back door). Left side—dining room. Right side—living room.

Center of foyer on west side—staircase to 2nd floor. Wood paneling on east side.

Overall view photos taken.

Foyer: red carpeting. Dresser-like table with 3 drawers. One chair, white.

A bloodstain noticed on carpet. Ph+ [tested positive to phenolphthalein test (which is a test for the presence of blood)]. 28 inches to east wall. 19 inches to center of wall.

Wood fragments, fibers, and hairs also observed on carpet. Did not collect.

Several fresh cut out areas on east side wooden panel. Paint chips on floor. Did not collect.

Blood spatter found on staircase. Ph+. Photo.

White thread-like material found. Photo. 2 pieces were collected and packaged.

The coroner's initial conclusion was that the manner of death was accidental, but he subsequently changed it to homicide. Defense attorneys strongly disagreed with the change, stating that it was a case of suicide because (1) gunshot residue was found on Clarkson's hands and (2) blood DNA on the gun's exterior and inside the barrel matched hers. Neither side disputed the fact that the gun was discharged inside her mouth.

Superior Court Judge Larry Paul Fidler ruled that the one thousand transcript pages of grand jury hearings should be made public. This became a contentious issue in late 2004 when defense attorney Bruce Cutler waved the five-volume transcript and bellowed, "This is poison! That's why the prosecution wants it out there. It's full of lies," while prosecutor Douglas Sortino, in turn, stated that an unbiased jury would still be found even if transcripts were released. A related dispute occurred when the issue of Phil Spector's celebrity arose. "We've had celebrity trials before. We've been able to get unbiased jurors before,"

Sortino said, and, in a written brief, argued that Spector was not as famous as some celebrities who had faced trial in Los Angeles, including O. J. Simpson and Robert Blake. He continued: "Nearly all of the hit records he produced were made in the 1960s and 1970s. It is likely that most people who came of age after that period have no idea of who he is and no current interest in what he has done."

But Spector's attorney Roger Rosen countered that his client "is certainly an international star. Whether he rises to the level of Mr. Blake or Mr. Simpson or [Michael] Jackson, he is an individual who is quite well recognized," and Cutler added, "[Spector] is a musical icon all over the world."[22]

The Associated Press and the *Los Angeles Times* both asked that the documents be released. The defense accused the organizations of seeking the transcripts only for commercial purposes. "They will go out and sell their newspapers," Rosen said. "But this will have an effect on Mr. Spector's life."

The judge responded, "There already has been a great deal of publicity." And attorney Susan Seager, representing the *Times* and the AP, stated, "The press and the public have the right to attend court proceedings and the press provides oversight, making sure the proceedings are conducted fairly."[23] In the end, the transcripts were made public.

According to the newly released grand jury transcripts, Spector at first told police he mistakenly shot Clarkson, though he later said she shot herself. Alhambra police officer Beatrice Rodriguez testified before the grand jury that Spector exclaimed at his residence, "What's wrong with you guys? What are you doing? I didn't mean to shoot her. It was an accident. I have an explanation for this."[24]

Other parts of the five volumes of grand jury transcripts contained testimony from police, from women who had reportedly been threatened by Spector, and from friends of the actress.

Fidler ruled that prosecutors could present evidence involving four incidents in which Spector allegedly pulled guns on women, but he refused to allow six other incidents to be cited. Defense attorney Cutler argued that none of the allegations was true and dismissed the women as celebrity-chasing "acolytes and gold diggers" out for publicity.[25]

In 2004 Spector and his attorney Robert Shapiro had an acrimonious split over legal fees. The following year, in a deposition regarding a civil suit against Shapiro, Spector revealed

> [t]hat for the previous eight years, he took daily doses of Prozac, Clonopin, Neurontonin—and two other medications he couldn't recall—to help relieve manic depression and symptoms he described as "sleeplessness, depression, mood changes, mood swings, hard to live with, hard to concentrate, hard—just hard—a hard time getting through life."
>
> That he may have once questioned his sanity with a reporter in jest, "because I've been called a genius and I think genius is not there all the time and has borderline insanity."
>
> That he had a son named Philip who died of leukemia at the age of ten.
>
> That he was engaged to a twenty-five-year-old model/actress named Rachelle Short.
>
> That when he was arrested, police officers on the scene Tasered and tackled him after he allegedly refused to follow their orders. Spector said he was later treated for a "broken septum" and a "cracked spine."
>
> That he was unaware Clarkson was dead until he was booked on suspicion of murder and heard a radio report about her death in the car after his release. "I know of my own knowledge she had been shot," he said, "but I didn't know that anybody had been—was—was dead."[26]

At a hearing in late 2005, Cutler tried desperately to dismiss all of Spector's comments on the night of the tragedy. Cutler insisted that most of the remarks were innocuous, though Spector reportedly said, "I'm sorry there's a dead woman here" and "If you're going to arrest me, just tell me what happened."

Cutler, who once represented Mob boss John Gotti, claimed that on the night of Clarkson's death, police "crashed" into Spector's home like "storm troopers," attacked him, hog-tied him, Tasered him, and "figuratively punched him around until he said something." He further held that the statements were inadmissible because the police had not read the producer his Miranda rights.[27]

Deputy District Attorney Douglas Sortino returned fire, saying there was no evidence of misconduct and noted that the Taser had no effect on the then sixty-four-year-old Spector, who had refused to come out of his house with his hands visible.

Fidler said the statements were definitely admissible because they were voluntarily offered. In addition, he said, Spector did not need to be Mirandized because he was never interrogated.

Cutler, his voice raised, said, "We deny in the clearest terms that he shot that lady." He pounded his fist on the dais. "We also deny in the clearest terms that Mr. Spector ever *admitted* that he shot that lady."[28]

And so it went, each of the forty-odd months filled with legal wrangling, maneuvering, accusations, counteraccusations, attorney resignations and firings, judicial rulings, and thinly veiled spin—both sides elbowing for the spotlight, jockeying for the best possible pretrial position. And all of it played out on a national stage.

THE TRIAL

Except for the verdict and a dramatic bombshell near the close of the defense's presentation, the trial was, in a sense, anticlimactic. The prosecution contended much of what it had already leaked to the public, all centered around a music legend-turned-recluse whose sexual advances had been spurned, the key testimony of his chauffeur, his previous history of gunplay, and the coroner's report. The defense focused on suicide as a manner of death, citing an aging actress who was despondent over a flagging Hollywood career and physical evidence from the death scene, such as blood spatter, gunshot residue, tissue residue, and the location of the wound.

A good deal of the five-month process of setting forth, examining, and deciding the case, however, was an intriguing lesson in strategy and tactics.

Opening Statements

In his opening statement to a jury of nine men and three women on April 25, 2007, Deputy District Attorney Alan Jackson promised to reveal "the Real Phil Spector" as a dangerous gun nut whose "very rich history of violence" culminated in the alleged murder of an actress in his Alhambra mansion.

"He put a loaded pistol in her mouth and shot her to death," the prosecutor said, adding that prosecutors would present blood spatter evidence indicating Spector was within three feet of the victim at the time of her death. He branded the shooting as "simply the last of a very long line of women who have been victimized by [him]," and stated that in each case, a drunken Spector pulled a weapon on a woman he was sexually interested in when she tried to leave his residence. What emerged, Jackson said, is a picture of Phil Spector as a man who, when confronted with the right circumstances, the right situation, "turn[ed] sinister and deadly."[29]

One mini-surprise unfolded on that first trial day when the prosecution opted to deviate from its expected strategy of introducing into evidence Spector's statements to police immediately after Clarkson was found dead. Some legal scholars later declared the move as either a tactical blunder or a blessing.

On the one hand, from the prosecution's perspective, it caught the defense completely off guard, for the statements had been the subject of that pretrial legal battle in 2005 when the prosecution prevailed in its quest to have them admissible. Furthermore, parts of the statements could have helped the defense in its theory that the actress took her own life—for example, Spector's statement to police officers: "And I don't know what her f—ing problem was, but she certainly had no right to come to my f—ing castle, blow her f—ing head open." On the other hand, the switch might have helped the defense more in the long run, for the statement "I think I killed somebody" certainly carried weight in the prosecution's favor.

The interesting point here is that both sides understood the California law that bars a defendant's admissions as hearsay unless introduced by the prosecution. Thus the prosecution held a trump card if it ever wanted to use it.

The switch also hurt the defense in another way. Cutler had already prepared his opening, based on his understanding that those statements would be heard by the jury. However, with the change, he would have to abandon his approach in favor of an extemporaneous, "from the hip" address. He said to Fidler that he had mapped his opening around the statements and suggested the defense had been misled by the prosecutors. He emphasized that his client's remarks on the night of the killing were consistent with a self-inflicted gunshot wound but that now, most of the remarks would not be allowed in.

"I feel like my pants are down and I am naked before the court," he complained to the judge. "I didn't know until just this moment that the prosecution team was not going to use the statements.... So [the] police are not going to testify about these things?"

"That's correct," Fidler replied.

"It's one-sided, your honor. It's completely unfair," Cutler grumbled.

"It's called the law," the judge snapped.[30]

And all the while, a conservatively dressed Phil Spector sat stone-faced, as he would for the duration of the trial.

Once it was clear that Cutler had to scrap his prepared opening remarks, he gave a less rousing address suggesting that police had rushed to judgment because of his client's wealth and fame.

The lead defense attorney was followed by attorney Linda Kenney-Baden, who was brought in to handle the forensic aspects of the case. She told the jury she could produce a witness with "no memory problems," no agendas, and no language barrier. "And that witness is called science," she said.

She indicated the defense would offer ten separate scientific bases on which it could be proven that Spector did not fire the shot. Among them was the small amount of blood spatter on the white coat the defendant was wearing in contrast to the extensive blood patterns on Clarkson's garments, chest, and face.

She said the same applied to brain tissue and gunshot residue—that brain tissue was detected on the buttons of Clarkson's sleeve but not on Spector's clothes, suggesting she had held her hands up to her mouth in pulling the trigger. "It proves scientifically that he, Philip, was not near her when she was shot."

With respect to gunshot residue, she stated the amount on Clarkson's clothing and body contrasted dramatically with what she said was a minimal amount on her client. She also stressed that DNA tests proved that Spector had not fired the gun. "They found only Lana Clarkson's DNA and some other unknown person's [on the gun], not Phil Spector's."[31]

Kenney-Baden read from some of Clarkson's e-mails in an effort to illustrate the actress's state of mind, her struggles to make ends meet, and her worries about the future:

> I'm going to tidy my affairs and chuck it because it is really too much for this girl to bear.

> Wish I was busier with fabulous paid acting work. Tons of follow up mailings and paper work to do, but the depression level I am experiencing due to major financial difficulties, makes me feel spent and worn out. I was to attend that party tonight and am instead going to stay home and veg, watching bad free library movies. I am looking into other gigs.... It's tuff to find a job these days.... I am so tired of struggling to eat! Anyway, I am normally such a happy positive person. Seems I am always in the dumps when you check in. Sorry about that.

I feel really bad taking you up on your offer of a $200.00 loan. I thought with all the hours you've been working and the fact that you have credit cards, that you in a more solid position. I certainly wouldn't want to [affect] your family holiday adversely in anyway. If you can do that, that'd be great. I would never have asked had you not offered. I have nowhere else to turn right now, as I mentioned last night. I will most probably have to move from the cottage, but this small loan will at least help in some way or another. . . . I am sorry not to telephone you tonight but this way you cannot hear my tears. I am truly at the end of this whole deal.

Well, I'm gonna hit the hay. I'm beat after tidying up my pad. I really trashed it in the midst of my depression. Trying to hold my head up high and know that God has many wonderful things in store for me. For us all!

Over here things are pretty bad. I won't go into detail but I am on the verge of losing it all. Just hanging on by a thread.[32]

Testimony for the Prosecution

The next day, the government opened its case with the testimony of the first of five ex-girlfriends who all claimed Spector menaced them with weapons under circumstances it contends resembled those in the Clarkson shooting. Such sworn statements along with (1) the testimony of Spector's chauffeur and (2) the issue of whether or not I had hidden certain evidence from the prosecution (see page 32)—filled the first month of the trial. This period—from approximately April 25 to May 25, 2007—represented half the time the prosecution required to present its entire case.

Selected incidents involving the five women were surprisingly similar.

Diane Ogden, a talent-casting coordinator, was the last guest at a dinner party Spector hosted in 1989. When she leaned over to kiss him good-bye, he brandished a rifle and screamed obscenities at her. He then got a handgun and pressed the nose of it against her face. He ordered her into his bed and attempted to have sexual intercourse with her, but did not.

"He was not my Phil. He wasn't the man I loved. I mean, I cared about this man, and it wasn't him. It was like he was demonic," Ogden said.

During a Fourth of July sleepover at Spector's home in 1993, Dorothy Melvin, former manager to comedienne Joan Rivers, fell asleep in his living room and awoke to find him outside pointing a gun at her brand-new Mercedes. When she refused his expletive-filled command to reenter the house, he struck her on the head with a snub-nosed revolver.

"I was sobbing," Melvin testified. "And I said, 'Why are you doing this, Phil? Why are you doing this?'"

At gunpoint he ordered her to undress. She eventually was allowed to leave. He followed her down his driveway, waving a shotgun at her.

"Phil is a very brilliant and charming man, and you really enjoy him when he is in his charming mode," she said, "but when he drinks, he snaps and he turns on a dime and becomes a lunatic."[33]

Spector put up waitress Melissa Grosvenor in a hotel near his home in 1992. At his place, following dinner at a restaurant, he pointed a handgun at her face while screaming profanities. She never dated him again but saw him on numerous occasions in the restaurant at which she worked. He asked her to come back to the hotel several times.

"I said 'no' and he threatened me and said, 'I've got machine guns and I know where you live,'" Grosvenor recalled.

Spector invited freelance photographer Stephanie Jennings to accompany him to an after-party for the Rock and Roll Hall of Fame induction ceremony in 1994, putting her up at the same upscale hotel where he had a suite. Later, while "extremely drunk," he ordered her to his bedroom. She refused and began packing to leave.

"He had a gun with him and he pulled a chair in front of the door and said I was not going anywhere," Jennings said. She called 911 and left unharmed.

Devra Robitaille, an administrative director for Warner-Spector Records, testified that one evening she was the last guest to leave his house. He was intoxicated. When she said she wanted to leave, he put a gun to her head and threatened to shoot her. Eventually she was allowed to leave.[34]

In calling the above string of women to the stand—all of whom had dated Spector in the 1980s and 1990s and recounted the rise and fall of their relationships with him—the prosecution hoped to paint the portrait of a music industry Dr. Jekyll and Mr. Hyde. Each, in her own way, described her reaction to his gun threats as equal parts terror and astonishment, because, each said, the threat came from a man as well known to them for his chivalrous kindness as he was for producing the work of such stars as the Beatles and Tina Turner.

During the course of their two weeks of testimony, jurors appeared fully absorbed by the women's stories. Loyola Law School professor Stanley Goldman observed: "Jurors take this kind of evidence and run with it. If he's done it before, they think, he's obviously done it now."

Goldman disagreed with trial judge Fidler's decision to admit past bad behavior by the defendant, because it has the effect of lowering the burden of proof (for the prosecution). "He's now defending [six] cases—the [five women] and what he's actually charged with," Goldman said.

Other legal analysts agreed that cross-examining the women proved to be a huge challenge (and a great opportunity) for the defense, in part because of the many positive things they said about the defendant. Defense attorneys in no way wanted to inhibit that aspect of the testimony. All of the women, for example, said they were testifying only because they had been subpoenaed by prosecutors, and some seemed torn about offering any evidence against Spector.[35]

In the third week of the trial, the defendant's chauffeur, Adriano DeSouza, spent four days on the witness stand. His statement, quoting Spector shortly after the shooting as saying, "I think I killed somebody," was repeated throughout his testimony—words that were so direct and incriminating, they became the cornerstone of the prosecution's case.

DeSouza said that when he first saw Spector exiting from the rear door of his mansion, the producer had a small black revolver in his right hand and some blood on his index finger. Peering around his employer's small frame and into the foyer, he observed the lifeless body of the actress slumped in a chair.

"I saw blood on her face," the thirty-seven-year-old chauffeur said.

A native of Brazil, DeSouza spoke with a thick accent as he recalled the various stops at West Hollywood and Beverly Hills restaurants on the night of February 2. As the evening drew on, he had noticed that Spector was becoming intoxicated.

Before Spector emerged, the chauffeur said, he had been parked outside the rear door listening to the radio for about two hours. Suddenly he heard a "pow," and very shortly thereafter, Spector appeared. He walked to a point within four to six feet of DeSouza.

"He was like a little bit slow, speaking slow, starting to have some difficulty to talk," DeSouza told the jury.

The defense had indicated earlier that the chauffeur did not speak English well enough to quote Spector accurately; specifically, Cutler suggested in his opening statement that the driver actually heard, "I think somebody is killed." And on his first day of testimony, DeSouza admitted he had trouble understanding the producer "when he was drunk."[36]

On the driver's second day of testimony—May 17, 2007—jurors heard his panicked 911 call. "I think my boss killed somebody," DeSouza told an emergency operator. "He have a lady on the, on the floor and he have a gun in his hand."

He explained he was so terrified by the scene that he momentarily forgot how to use his cell phone and fled on foot away from Spector before hopping in his boss's car and speeding outside the gates of the estate. There he placed two calls: the first to Spector's assistant, Michelle Blaine, because he needed to learn the street address before calling the police through 911.

Blaine did not answer, so he left a voicemail message that was also played for the jury: "You have to come to Mr. Philip's house. I think he killed some—please call me, call me back now."

Under intense cross-examination by defense attorney Bradley Brunon, which lasted more than two hours, DeSouza said he had been in the United States on a student visa for four years and acknowledged the visa did not allow him to work in this country.

"So you didn't respect the law that allows you to come here?" Brunon asked.

"Uh, no," the driver responded.

Brunon then turned to the issue of Spector's voice, specifically its soft-spoken quality. The lawyer asked the witness to describe the defendant's voice.

"I am not good at describe voices," DeSouza said. "If you want me to talk like him—" He then gave a whining, high-pitched imitation of his boss, saying, "Adriano, Adriano..." Courtroom spectators erupted in laughter. But Spector remained impassive.

Accusation Most Foul

This was also the day when I was mortified to hear in open court about a ridiculous charge leveled at me by a former defense attorney on the case. It had been raised before—two weeks earlier—at a special hearing before Fidler, but it had also surfaced as an allegation of missing evidence—without names mentioned—just after Clarkson's death in 2003. At the time, defense attorney Robert Shapiro assured a judge that nothing had been held back from prosecutors, and within a year, the issue was put to rest.

At the special hearing, two former insiders on the defense team, attorney Sara Caplan and private investigator Stanley White, told the judge that I had concealed evidence recovered from the death scene. I have a one-word response to such an accusation: Preposterous!

Caplan, a former associate of Shapiro's, stated she saw me pluck "a little white thing"—about one inch long—from the foyer and place it in a clear evidence vial, but that such evidence was never turned over to authorities. She said she did not know what became of the object, which she described as "flat with uneven edges" and about the size of a fingernail. "I didn't watch what he did with that," she said, referring to me.

White, a former Los Angeles detective, said he was present when I announced finding human "tissue" and indicated he had a short but vehement disagreement with me about what the item was.

White stated: "I said it looked like a piece of fingernail. Dr. Lee said to me, 'You're crazy.' I said back, 'You need glasses.'"

At the risk of convoluting this issue, I must point out that there had actually been *three* days of hearings and witnesses—with Fidler, but outside the presence of the jury. During that stretch of time, Fidler said he wanted to hear directly from me, but, as it so happened, I was in Italy, lecturing at the University of Verona Medical School. I read later that the judge declared, "I believe the court has an absolute obligation when there is any inference or allegation that any evidence has been tampered with to make inquiry.... We now have to continue to guarantee the sanctity of any evidence or lack of evidence that may be presented to the court."[37]

In the same week as the special hearings, my colleague Dr. Michael Baden was brought into the picture when a former law clerk, Gregory Diamond, claimed he saw members of the defense team find what the famed forensic pathologist identified as *possibly* a tooth fragment that had been overlooked by crime scene technicians.

It is revealing to make mention of the several inconsistencies in the above three accounts.

Diamond testified that I never handled the object. He stated it was Caplan, in fact, who had picked it up off the carpet and Baden who examined it.

Caplan denied ever touching it and said White could not have seen me handling anything because he was consigned to guard duty outside the mansion and never entered the foyer.

To be clear on this issue, the object in question that both Baden and Caplan together found on the carpet and an object I *allegedly* handled (but did not) were one and the same.

Bill Pavelic, a well-known private investigator, had also been at the scene and, testifying for the defense, took the stand before White and Caplan. He stated he never saw me or anyone else touch a small white piece of evidence, much less collect it into an evidence vial. When asked about White, Pavelic scoffed, "I consider Mr. White to be a prosecution witness and a snitch."[38]

There was another special hearing during that second day of DeSouza's testimony, May 17. When asked whether I had seen or recovered a piece of fingernail during a defense search of the shooting scene, I answered, "Definitely not." I then hinted that what Caplan thought were vials were actually plastic reagent tubes used for blood testing.

"I think she made an honest mistake," I said. But I was also quick to state, "I think my reputation [is] severely damaged."[39]

And while we're on the subject of attacks on my credibility—the first time in my forty-five years as a forensic scientist—I should bring up two other things.

First, in an April 2007 interview on Court TV, I stated that blood spatter could be expected to travel seventy-two inches from a gunshot wound such as the one suffered by Lana Clarkson. This statement was included in the defense's opening statement the next day. By then the prosecution's opening statement had concluded. So what did the prosecution claim? That Spector's defense team had deliberately violated rules for sharing evidence and should be sanctioned by the judge.

Second, Caplan had refused to testify about the white object issue. Fidler promised to have her jailed if she failed to cooperate. The state supreme court rejected her appeal of contempt of court charges. The upshot is that she finally took the witness stand and, under questioning by the defense, said that the item I placed in a vial was too big to be a chip from Clarkson's acrylic thumbnail, as the prosecution had suggested.

"You are sure that what you saw was much larger than that missing piece of fingernail?" she was asked.

"I am sure," she replied.

She said that while she could not say what the object was, it was an inch long, the size of an "entire fingernail" and not the fragment missing from Clarkson's thumbnail. "It could have been something someone dragged in on their foot," she added.[40]

In the final analysis of this phase of the case, University of Southern California law professor Jean Rosenbluth commented, "Although he implied it, [Fidler] didn't make a finding that Henry Lee lied on the stand and he didn't make a finding that he acted maliciously."

As for the residual effect on my reputation, I must say that I can live with my conscience. I didn't even know a fingernail was broken and I didn't find a fingernail. You know, when they can't destroy the science, they try to destroy your reputation.

The last two days of the chauffeur's testimony centered primarily on painstaking cross-examination by the defense. Such questioning, in turn, was concerned with DeSouza's grasp of English, whether or not he heard Spector correctly on that early morning of the killing, and the driver's desire to avoid being deported because of immigration violations.

To bolster the possibility that what he really heard Spector say differed from what he had told authorities, defense lawyer Brunon noted that the chauffeur had not slept in twenty-four hours, that he was frightened by the shooting, that Spector was drunk and perhaps slurring his words, and that the sound of a large fountain may have interfered with DeSouza's hearing. All in all, however, DeSouza stuck to the central claim that, despite these factors, he had heard Spector utter, "I think I killed somebody."

As damaging to the defense as that one sentence was, the testimony of the coroner was at least as damaging. Dr. Louis Pena, the deputy coroner who had examined Clarkson's body and performed the autopsy, injected the most direct "scientific" approach to the prosecution's case. Until then, the Los Angeles District Attorney's Office had tried to build a case on a pattern of booze, guns, and past violence against women.

Pena testified that there were bruises on the victim's right arm and wrist, which he called "resistance injuries." The implication was that the bruises were not indicative of someone who grabbed a gun and shot herself, but rather of someone who fought with an assailant who was trying to kill her. What's more, there was a bruise on her tongue consistent with someone having shoved a gun into her mouth.

"The bruise is very unique," he said, "and is consistent with blunt-force trauma. Something struck the tongue."

The coroner offered other reasons why he arrived at the conclusion that the death was a homicide, testifying that:

- There was no blood in the crevices of the gun, implying that it had been wiped clean after the shooting. "This tells me someone manipulated the gun," he said.
- The victim was a hopeful person, working regularly and socializing with friends. Also, she had made no effort to get any affairs in order before she died, not typical of one contemplating suicide, in his opinion.
- Clarkson's purse was found draped over her right shoulder. She was right-handed. He said that if she was planning to shoot herself, the "purse should have been taken off and dropped."
- The location of the death was an unlikely one for suicide. He said people usually commit suicide in private, not at the home of another person, especially not someone they had just met.
- The actress had never been in the home before, and investigators did not find multiple drawers in the house pulled open. Only the drawer in the foyer—the one with the holster—was found open. He stated, "I've never seen a case reported in which somebody enters a stranger's house and magically comes up with a gun and shoots herself. How would she have known where the gun is?"[41]
- She had no history of major depression or previous psychiatric disorder. He said two medications she was taking were prescribed to her by a neurologist treating her for recurrent headaches. If she had planned to kill herself, he opined, she could have overdosed rather than using a gun.

Under cross-examination, Pena said he initially ruled the death an accident but subsequently as a homicide after examining reports of investigators and other materials related to the case, a process he conceded he rarely did in his work at the coroner's office.

"This is kind of new to me," he admitted.

The defense used the admission to launch into Pena's inexperience in this area of pathology. It touched on the relative rarity of the type of injury Clarkson suffered, known as "intra-oral gunshot wound." When asked, Pena said he had seen only one other case in the thirty-three hundred autopsies he had performed in his career. He acknowledged that he had relied on textbooks written by Dr. Vincent Di Maio and Dr. Werner Spitz, two forensic pathologists hired by the defense.

The cross-examination lasted three days, during which time Pena did not budge from his conclusion that Clarkson was murdered. Yet he seemed to sidestep—or rationalize away—the issue of her mental state in the weeks and months preceding her death. And the defense took advantage of that tactic, likely wanting to raise doubts about the pathologist's preparation before rendering a decision regarding the manner of death.

When queried about a Web page bookmarked on her computer about screening for alcohol dependency and depression, for example, he responded, "I would have looked into that. It was not provided to me."[42]

After hearing some of Clarkson's e-mails read into evidence, Pena declared he had not known the extent of her financial problems or that she was seeking loans from a friend. But he said the e-mails seemed to reveal "situational" negative feelings, not clinical depression.

The next day, jurors were shown an array of items seized from Spector's mansion. Los Angeles sheriff's detective Mark Lillienfeld, who had supervised the collection of evidence, took the stand. Lillienfeld testified that an empty liter of tequila was found on a coffee table in the living room. Nearby was a brandy snifter, half full with an unidentified type of liquor. There was a second snifter resting on a sink in a powder room off the foyer. A pair of false eyelashes was also found in that room. Witnesses had previously said that Spector was drunk, while tests of Clarkson's blood showed an alcohol level of 0.12, above the legal limit to drive.

Lillienfeld said he found a "three-pack" of Viagra in a leather briefcase on a chair just a few feet from the body. "PS" was engraved on the briefcase. Two of the pills were gone from the pack. It should be noted that driver DeSouza had previously testified that Spector came out of the house to retrieve the briefcase from his Mercedes shortly after he and Clarkson entered the house.

Much of the detective's testimony dealt with guns and ammunition recovered from the house, including the Colt Cobra revolver that allegedly was the death weapon. Displaying it before the jury, he said it was found near Clarkson's right hand. She was right-handed. Lillienfeld stated he recalled seeing wet blood on the grip of the gun. And, of course, he drew attention to the holster in the partially opened drawer.

When asked about the number of phones throughout the mansion, the witness said he located more than a dozen, including a landline and two cell phones just a few steps from Clarkson's body. The point made here was that Spector did not phone 911 for help after the shooting.

Another prosecution witness, criminalist Steve Renteria of the Los Angeles County Sheriff's Department, testified that DNA found on Clarkson's wrists was consistent with Phil Spector's. He added that DNA taken from the two brandy snifters and from two drinking glasses was consistent with both Spector's and Clarkson's, a finding that indicated they had been sharing drinks.

The location of blood in the foyer was brought up by the prosecution. The defense had maintained all along that Spector was not close enough to Clarkson to have fired the gun in her mouth. The question of how far the blast from a gun can propel a victim's blood is one I would have answered had I testified. My answer—as far as six feet—would have been based on several factors, including the size of the blood drops. In general, big drops, having more mass, can overcome air resistance, so they can travel a fairly great distance, but as they move through the air they break up into mistlike droplets. In addition, the wound that occurs when a bullet enters the mouth (intra-oral gunshot wound) results in a powerful explosion of gases, leading to back spatter that could travel farther than one might expect.

The following day, Renteria, who indicated that he had worked with

DNA analysis since 1994, said he found Spector's DNA on Clarkson's left breast and a "very weakly positive" genetic profile of Clarkson on Spector's genitals. He also testified that Spector's DNA was not present on any part of the Colt handgun, on the bullets within the weapon, or under the victim's broken fingernail. And there was no indication of assault or sexual intercourse. The lack of DNA on the gun raised some questions about what the chauffeur had seen at Spector's house. He had testified that he saw the record producer emerge from the house holding a bloody gun and declaring, "I think I killed somebody." But the gun was found near Clarkson's right hand. More than one observer noted that such conflicting accounts of where the gun actually was—in the defendant's hand or near the victim's hand—would not eliminate the possibility that Clarkson did indeed pull the trigger. It should also be mentioned that it is not uncommon for a person to use *both* hands in an intra-oral type of suicide shooting.

Furthermore, absence of Spector's DNA from under Clarkson's fingernail would support the defense's theory that there had been no struggle between the pair before the shooting.

In cross-examination, Christopher Plourd, a defense attorney extremely knowledgeable in the area of forensic evidence, asked the criminalist to elaborate on the DNA found on Spector's body. Renteria stated that the DNA from the victim's breast matched the defendant's, and that the match could be expected in one in every 14.8 billion Caucasians. The profile on Spector's genitals was more common, he said: One in 94,000 Caucasians share it.

He also talked about tests performed on the grip of the revolver: Clarkson's DNA was present on several areas of the gun; Spector's was not.

"[T]hese markers are consistent with her and inconsistent with Mr. Spector, is that correct?" Plourd asked.

"Yes," Renteria replied.

But later, the prosecution—resorting to the old trick about the absence of evidence not meaning evidence of absence—said that the presence of a large amount of Clarkson's blood on the gun may have hidden Spector's DNA.

"You cannot exclude Philip Spector?" asked prosecution attorney Alan Jackson.

"Correct, or any other male," Renteria responded.[43]

The prosecution rested its case—at least temporarily—on June 22, 2007. It would be a month before it actually wrapped up its case. The "overlap" was caused by the issue of the so-called missing piece of evidence (the alleged "little white thing" I supposedly found, which was alluded to before). Fidler had allowed prosecutors to leave their case open as attorney Caplan fought the order to testify against me. After the state supreme court turned down her appeal, she agreed to take the witness stand, where she emphasized that "the little white thing" was *not* a fingernail.

On June 22, the last day of the first phase of the prosecution's case, Dr. Lynn Herold took the stand. The senior criminalist in the sheriff's department, Herold stated that the tiny red spots on the sleeves and lapels of Spector's white jacket indicated that he was standing within three feet of the deceased when she was shot (a point many bloodstain experts would dispute).

She also told jurors that blood had been "moved or removed" from the Colt revolver between its firing and the time police recovered it.

"Could that be the result of someone...wiping the gun down?" Jackson asked.

"That is one possible mechanism," Herold said.

On cross-examination, Kenney-Baden suggested that Herold was biased and also inexperienced in analyzing bloodstain patterns. The attorney noted that Herold's primary responsibilities at the crime lab ranged from examining hairs, fibers, and shoeprints to determining a deceased person's stomach contents.

Herold defended her experience in blood pattern analysis, citing her role in about one hundred such examinations in a twenty-five-year career. She admitted, however, that Clarkson's case was the first one in which she was asked to interpret stains from an intra-oral gunshot wound.[44]

Testimony for the Defense

The defense opened its case on June 28, 2007, with the testimony of Dr. Vincent Di Maio, a world-renowned gunshot wound expert and medical examiner. He said in no uncertain terms that "objective scientific evidence" indicated Clarkson's death was not a case of murder—that blood and gunshot residue on her hands convinced him the gunshot was self-inflicted.

"There is no objective scientific evidence that anyone else held the gun. Everything else is speculative," he said.

He brushed off allegations by prosecution investigators and statements by Spector's chauffeur as "speculating about what people said, what people did, what people felt." He then leaned toward the jury, lowered his voice to a whisper, and, as if sharing a secret, said, "Anything could be anything, but when you stick to the objective scientific facts, it is a suicide."

Readjusting himself in the witness chair, the pathologist, nationally renowned for his textbook on gunshot wounds, then commented on a list of forensic issues as if they were articles of faith:

- That in his thirty-eight years of experience as a pathologist, he had learned that "people do not want to accept suicides so they will try to make suicides into homicides."
- That large amounts of gunshot residue on Clarkson's hands contrasted sharply with the single particle recovered from Spector's hands. "The person who has abundant particles is most consistent with having the gun, not the person with one particle," he contended.
- That the blood spatter on Clarkson's hands was the suicide equivalent of a positive pregnancy test. "It is not always present," he said, "but if it is there, it is there."
- That certain statistics supported suicide, saying that 87 percent of women who kill themselves do so by shooting themselves, with 76 percent of them firing into their heads, and that in his experience, 99 percent of intra-oral gunshots point to suicide.[45]

On the second of his three days of testimony, Di Maio—arguably the most potent defense witness—endured a blistering cross-examination by Jackson. But the forensic pathologist never budged in his claim that Clarkson committed suicide.

When accused of misleading the jury about the significance of gunshot residue evidence, he shouted, "I told the truth!"

He contradicted the coroner's conclusion that the bruise on Clarkson's tongue was caused by Spector's shoving the revolver into her mouth. The pathologist called such a theory "impossible" given the anatomy of the mouth, and he attributed the bruise to the force of gases exploding as she pulled the trigger.

He referred to the actress's dwindling prospects in Hollywood and to her being a depressed, destitute woman with drug and alcohol problems—all corroborated by e-mails and other evidence from her personal computer.

"She was an actress who was forty years of age. I'm sorry. It's sex discrimination but that's the way it is," he said with a shrug.

He dismissed the prosecution's theory that the muzzle of the Colt revolver blew off a piece of Clarkson's acrylic fingernail as she tried to push the gun out of her mouth. He maintained that it was instead knocked off by the weapon's recoil, and, what's more, that if her finger had been inside her mouth, the blast would have melted the nail and left her other fingers "covered with blood, soot, powder and tissue." The finger, the doctor stressed, was "pristine."

He concluded his second day of testimony using a clear plastic model of Clarkson's head, and in so doing offered an explanation of how Clarkson held the gun. (The prosecution previously revealed it was unable to determine from blood evidence the position of her hands at the time of the shot.) Di Maio said that blood spots led him to conclude that her hands were wrapped around the gun grip with her thumbs on the trigger.[46]

The better part of the pathologist's last day of testimony concerned the actress's state of mind and the thinking—or lack of it—that possibly led to a decision to commit suicide. He said hers was not a typical suicide, but rather an "impulsive" one fueled by alcohol use and depression. He stated it involved no planning but was a spur-of-the-moment decision Clarkson made after consuming what he said were a half dozen drinks.

"This is an impulsive action with no thought of the consequences," is the way he expressed it.

He added, "She's a very beautiful girl, but she's forty years old and there are plenty of twenty-year-old girls after the parts she is after.... She is competing against Paris Hilton and things like that."

Jackson accused Di Maio of "cherry-picking" details of Clarkson's life but ignoring Spector's past history.

The pathologist said he considered their backstories a "wash" when it came to deciphering what he called "the question of this trial: who fired the gun?"

And he probably best summarized what he had been insisting all along when he testified, "There [are] things against Mr. Spector. There are things against Ms. Clarkson. In the end, you sit there and say you can't decide, so you have to go with the physical evidence."[47]

The second phase of the prosecution's overlapping presentation featured Rich Tomlin, the detective who led the investigation into Clarkson's death. He testified I had never handed over to him a small, white solid item about the size of a thumbnail. Although the issue of the so-called missing evidence had occupied many days of court time since the trial began, the vast majority of it had played out at special hearings outside the jury's presence. And until Tomlin's testimony, only two of the government's thirty-five witnesses had mentioned such an object.

Returning to the case for the defense, a second high-profile forensic pathologist, Dr. Werner Spitz, took the stand and echoed much of what Di Maio had said. Spitz agreed with his colleague's opinion of how Clarkson held the revolver, adding that he found the coroner's homicide ruling hasty and erroneous—that Clarkson had, in fact, died by her own hands. Like Di Maio, he quoted statistics and cited some of Clarkson's writings to buttress his conclusion. He emphasized that the type of injury Clarkson suffered is almost never homicide, and that, in his fifty-four-year career and in the performance or supervision of some sixty thousand autopsies, he had never encountered such a wound that turned out to be murder. He recounted his experience as a medical examiner in Michigan and Maryland and his role as an expert to two committees looking into the assassination of President John F. Kennedy.

When reminded of Spector's previous behavior toward women, he retorted, "What occurred ten or twelve or fifteen years earlier has little, if anything, to do with what happened on that day . . . in the presence of the scientific findings which require no other interpretation."

He said his ruling of suicide was based primarily on physical evidence at the death scene, including an absence of blood, tissue, and gunpowder on Spector's pants and shoes. He conceded that small droplets of blood on the defendant's evening jacket were likely spatter from the gunshot blast, but that Spector could have been standing up to six feet away at the time (echoing my opinion).

Jackson responded sarcastically, "Mr. Spector was so unlucky that he happened to be standing in the one spot six feet away, that every single impact spatter hit him, and nothing hit the ground in front of him, nothing."

Spitz's response was immediate. "When you say all of that, it sounds like you have a bucket of [blood]," he said, then joked that the line of questioning reminded him of the "magic bullet" theory in the Kennedy assassination.

As was the case in the cross-examination of Di Maio, the prosecution attempted to portray Spitz as a hired gun, referring to his handsome daily fee as a defense witness.[48] This is an issue that is regularly raised by the prosecution in most trials; prosecutors never seem to ask their own expert witnesses about being paid, either by the government or through consulting fees.

The remainder of the defense's case involved a succession of witnesses whose testimony lasted about a month. Among them was Spector's daughter, Nicole. She testified that her father is right-handed, a fact supporting defense's contention that it likely ruled out her father as the shooter, according to testimony by blood spatter experts, because Clarkson's blood was found on the left side of his jacket.

From that point on, key elements up to and including closing arguments were as follows:

- The "Baden Blockbuster." My close colleague Dr. Michael Baden electrified the courtroom when he posited an unanticipated theory about the origin of Clarkson's blood on Spector's jacket. He said it was possible that Clarkson did not die immediately from her injury but that she lived several minutes afterward, during which time she coughed up blood onto the jacket. This idea would be supported by fellow pathologist Spitz, who later returned to the witness stand. Both the prosecution and Fidler expressed outrage at the last-minute, previously unshared hypothesis. The defense had not informed the prosecution of the new theory—as is required by law—and Fidler ruled that the defense had violated discovery laws, which require both sides to notify each other of evidence in advance.
- Spector waived his right to testify in the trial.
- Cutler resigned from the case after hearing he would not be delivering a closing argument. Spector explained that the lawyer had had frequent clashes with and unfair treatment by Fidler, had taken several extended leaves of absence from the case, and may have lost some credibility with the jury.[49]
- In a special hearing attended by both sides but not the jury panel, the judge ruled that jury members would have only one question to decide: Is the defendant guilty or not guilty of second-degree murder? In other words, manslaughter or other lesser charges would not be an option. He indicated that Spector had been charged with second-degree murder under a theory known as "implied malice." Thus prosecutors were not required to prove that he shot Clarkson deliberately, only that he was behaving with a conscious disregard for human life when he killed her. Fidler

made clear that placing a loaded handgun in a person's mouth would qualify as "conscious disregard for human life," even if that weapon discharged accidentally.

- In response to Fidler's ruling, Jackson said, "She could have slapped his hand and it could have gone off. He could have sneezed and it could have gone off."[50]
- In the prosecution's four-hour closing argument, Jackson painted Spector as a violent misogynist who shot Lana Clarkson because she rejected the Viagra-fueled sexual encounter he had planned. "He had one thing on his mind," he said, "[and] she had another." He referenced earlier testimony that Spector referred to women by a profane term and had once said, "[A]ll deserve a bullet in their heads." Jackson commented, "That is Phil Spector's mindset. Women are all f—ing c-words." He played a video montage of the testimony of the five women who claimed Spector had threatened them with weapons over the past three decades. He noted similarities to Clarkson's death and said that perhaps a more apt confession by Spector would have been, "I think I *finally* killed somebody." Jackson labeled the evidence presented by the Spector team a "checkbook defense," saying of defense witnesses, both expert and lay, "It's nothing more than a pay to say. If you pay it, I will say it....If you hire enough lawyers who hired enough experts who are paid enough money, you can get them to say just about anything."[51]
- (To those who question the fees of such experts, investigative journalist Dawna Kaufmann has responded: "Like defense experts who command a high price for their services, government witnesses are also well paid, and their services include health insurance and retirement benefits which are funded by taxpayers.")[52]
- The defense, in the person of Linda Kenney-Baden, presented a six-hour closing argument. In it, she charged that law enforcement officials railroaded Spector because they were desperate to win a conviction against a celebrity: "They had a history of high-profile cases [e.g., O. J. Simpson and Robert Blake] and a history

of bad results." She implied that the legendary music producer would be the "first celebrity notch in the government's gun belt." She spent considerable time on the forensic evidence she said exonerated Spector, concentrating on the producer's dinner jacket and calling it "probably the most important piece of evidence" in the trial.

• She challenged the prosecution's claim that Spector was within three feet of Clarkson when the gun was fired, stating rather that the blast had propelled blood and tissue from her mouth and nose "like a bazooka." Asserting that the sleeves of Spector's white jacket would have been heavily stained had he been holding the Colt revolver in her mouth when it discharged, she said, "[T]hose areas were pristine."

• As for Spector's location at the time of the shooting, the defense attorney referred to the upward angle of the gunshot wound and said that, given the deceased's seated position in a low chair, "Philip Spector would have to be kneeling between her legs to get that angle ... he's short, ladies and gentlemen, but he is not that short."

• Finally, she dismissed the testimony of the five women and their claims against her client with the compelling statement: "Stories don't trump science."[53]

Two days later, jury deliberations began. They lasted forty-four hours over twelve days before Fidler declared a mistrial. A week before, the jury foreman had reported a seven-to-five split and Fidler withdrew a jury instruction that he decided had misstated the law. He substituted a new one, which included the possibility that Spector had forced Clarkson herself to insert the gun in her mouth. And almost another week later, the jury reported it was helplessly deadlocked, ten to two, in favor of conviction.

"The defense definitely dodged a bullet," said Stanley Goldman, the Loyola Law School professor who had publicly commented on the case earlier. "The reinstruction last week was definitely the judge nudging the jury toward finding Spector guilty."[54]

In writing about the verdict, Dan Glaister of the United Kingdom's *Guardian* newspaper focused not on Spector but on the struggles of a would-be starlet, and in so doing offered a unique perspective on the entire case:

> Two images of Lana Clarkson endure after the trial. In photograph after photograph displayed on an overhead projector in the courtroom, the actor, children's entertainer and nightclub hostess was shown in a series of coquettish poses: smiling at awards ceremonies or with friends at parties, she was the embodiment of the blonde, leggy starlet she dreamed of being.
>
> The other image, shown almost as frequently during the trial, was of her dead body slumped at an awkward angle in an ornate chair in the lobby of Spector's mansion, handbag hanging from her shoulder.
>
> Despite the graphic images, the real Clarkson remained an obscure figure during the trial. She was depressed, she took pharmaceutical drugs, she liked to drink, she knew how to ride horses, she had handled firearms. She was also desperate for success, looking for ways to relaunch her career as she entered her 40's. Did all this make her likely to commit suicide as the defense insisted? Or was she the determined professional the prosecution sought to depict? Ultimately the jury could not decide.[55]

My feeling about the trial is that it went counter to what I have always believed is at the core of the American justice system: a sense of fairness and truth. It appears to me that a full 162 days of trial consisted of little more than attacks on the victim, attacks on the suspect, and attacks on defense witnesses. Especially galling were references that expert defense witnesses were all "hired guns." The amount of time and money the prosecution expended in trying to dig up "some dirt" by checking educational backgrounds, income tax reports, and other personal affairs far exceeded what was necessary to unearth the facts—to seek the truth.

THE RETRIAL

A retrial got under way a little over a year after the jury was unable to reach a unanimous decision, and more than five years after Clarkson was found dead.

Law professor Jean Rosenbluth said she expected it to be shorter and more "streamlined" than the first. "For a start, each side has seen the other's presentation of evidence so they aren't going to be surprised," she said. "Both sides know what's coming and they're going to have thought ahead on how to counter it.... [The defense knows] what holes the prosecution were able to poke into them the first time around so they'll be much more focused.... [I]t will be streamlined because less people care. The world is not going to be watching as much as they were the first time."[56]

The latter assessment turned out to be correct; there was a sharp decline in public interest shortly after the deadlocked first trial, and the retrial was played out in a sparsely populated courtroom with few members of the media in attendance.

There was one procedural difference in the two trials. Jurors in the second one—in contrast to the first—were given the option of convicting Spector of involuntary manslaughter rather than the more serious offense of second-degree murder.

Some definitions are in order. "Murder" is the crime of intentionally killing someone, whereas "manslaughter" is killing through criminal negligence. First-degree murder is murder with malice aforethought; second-degree murder is murder in the heat of passion. Malice aforethought is the intent on the part of the defendant to harm someone before committing the act with which he or she has been charged. The negligence associated with manslaughter may be accidental or otherwise without malice. It may be voluntary or involuntary. Voluntary manslaughter is the crime of killing someone when provoked and in a highly distraught state; involuntary manslaughter is the killing of someone as a result of negligence, such as by causing a fatal automobile accident.

Several major players returned for the retrial, but some were new to the case.

Superior Court Judge Larry Fidler continued on as the presiding judge despite claims by Spector's legal team that he was clearly biased against the defendant. They cited his rulings toward the end of the first trial; for example, the defense insisted that the judge's "reinstruction" to the jury panel stating that Spector had possibly forced Clarkson to insert the gun into her mouth was designed to ensure a conviction. This tied into another factor, which many observers believed was pervasive throughout the year before the retrial even began. They were convinced that Fidler and the prosecutors—*all* prosecutors in the area—were still haunted by the past acquittals of celebrities such as O. J. Simpson, Michael Jackson, and the actor Robert Blake. Thus there was a feeling floating in and out of the courtroom that this time around, history would not repeat itself.

Deputy District Attorney Alan Jackson again headed up the prosecution's case. Most of the prosecution's testimony was a duplication of that in the initial trial. Once again a key witness was the chauffeur, Adriano DeSouza, who, the prosecution alleged, heard a gunshot just before he saw Spector emerge from his mansion and heard him say, "I think I killed somebody." And, as in the first trial, they presented testimony from five women who told of having been threatened by a drunken, gun-wielding Spector. The prosecution also contended that blood spatter evidence proved that Clarkson could not have shot herself.

But it was Deputy District Attorney Truc Do who provided the most dramatic moments of the retrial when, in her closing argument, she referred to the defendant as a "demonic maniac" when he drank and as "a very dangerous man" around women. "This case is about a man who had a history of playing Russian roulette with the lives of women," she said. "Five women got the empty chamber. Lana got the sixth bullet."[57]

Widely considered an expert in electronic evidence displays, Do projected a scene of dunes in her native Vietnam and said it illustrated the "shifting sands" of the defense team. She suggested evidence of Spector's washing his hands and attempting to wash blood from the victim's face after the shooting. "He can wash his hands clean of her blood," she said, "but he can't wash them clean of her murder."[58]

Spector's defense in the retrial was led by attorney Doron Weinberg. The team stressed that the chauffeur DeSouza, a Brazilian immigrant, was not fully proficient in English and said he might have misquoted Spector. They stated Spector might have said, "Call somebody." They also suggested that a gurgling fountain nearby might have interfered with the chauffeur's hearing, and that hunger and fatigue from working all night might have added to his confusion.

In closing arguments, Weinberg listed fourteen points of forensic evidence, including blood spatter, DNA, and gunshot residue, which he maintained were proof of a self-inflicted wound. "It's very difficult to put a gun into somebody's mouth," he told the jury. "Every single fact says this is a self-inflicted gunshot wound. How do you ignore it? How do you say this could have been homicide?"[59]

Finally, the jury of six men and six women ended the five-month-long retrial, reaching its decision after twenty-seven hours of deliberation, handing down the verdict of second-degree murder. In addition they found the defendant guilty of illegally discharging a firearm. Spector showed no emotion as the verdict was read, but his wife, Rachelle, sobbed. Fidler denied bail, and Spector was immediately remanded into custody to await sentencing six weeks later. On May 29, 2009, he was given a sentence of nineteen years to life and was told that he would not be eligible for parole until 2028, when he would be eighty-eight.

Weinberg's reaction to the verdict was to claim that the jury had been swayed by the testimony of the five women from Spector's past, that it was inappropriate for Fidler to have allowed such testimony to be introduced, and that it would be the basis for appeal and a request for yet another trial.[60]

Although this case may not be as sensational as, say, the O. J. Simpson or JonBenet Ramsey cases, it raises questions about credibility within, and even the basic spirit of, the American criminal justice system. From a legal perspective, for example, did the prosecution prove guilt beyond a reasonable doubt? Possibly. From a scientific perspective, however, many observers feel the evidence did *not* prove guilt beyond a reasonable doubt.

In a March 29, 2009, *Los Angeles Times* editorial titled "Spector—and Expert Witnesses—on Trial," it was suggested that prosecutorial witnesses are knowledgeable, above reproach, and without "bias." This, it claimed, is in contrast to defense witnesses.[61] But the editorial completely ignored the recent findings of the National Academy of Sciences, which addressed "the dismal quality of work produced by [most] crime labs throughout the United States." The academy's report indicated that scientific objectivity is routinely sacrificed to the perceived needs of law enforcement, and provided several hundred examples— and in the Spector case more than a dozen—of crime lab scientists' tailoring their findings to fit the theories of police officers and prosecutors. It specifically criticized government witnesses for bias and "junk science" testimony.

According to another *Los Angeles Times* editorial, the Spector record reveals that "from the moment police officers and their scientific experts arrived at the [Spector crime] scene, they alone determined what evidence was significant and what was not, what evidence should be tested and what should not, and what evidence should be seized and what should not."[62]

The reader may want to take another look at the scientific evidence and ask whether guilt, in this case, was proven beyond a reasonable doubt.

2

BROWN'S
CHICKEN MASSACRE

We move now to Chicago, a city once associated with prolific organized crime activity and higher than average crime rates, particularly during the Prohibition years. One of the grisliest mass murders in US history occurred there in 1993, but its victims were not Mob bosses or hoodlums. They were instead seven innocent, hard-working individuals, none of whom had ever been associated with bootlegging, loan-sharking, extortion, drug trafficking, prostitution, or Mob hits.

BACKGROUND

To get a better grasp on the sheer brutality of the Brown's Chicken massacre, an act committed not in retaliation—one Mob against another—but for reasons that even today remain difficult to compre-hend, we will first take a look back at Chicago's violent gangland past. In no city did rival gangs carry on such murderous assaults and coun-terassaults during Prohibition as they did in Chicago. Organized crime originated there in the 1870s, but it was not until the Roaring Twenties that it reached its heyday. This was in no small part due to various crime figures with nicknames like "Big Jim," "Bugs," "Bozo," "Crane Neck," "Schemer," "The Scourge," and "Hymie." It was Earl "Hymie" Weiss who coined the phrase "taking him for a ride"—a one-way ride.

But none measured up to "The Big Fellow"—Al Capone, perhaps the country's best-known gangster and a unique symbol of the collapse of law and order during the Prohibition era. It was the scope of his criminality and his violence that lent Chicago its reputation as a lawless city, a "wide-open town."

Those were the days of speakeasies, the Charleston, short skirts, rolled silk stockings, bobbed hair, raccoon coats, and blaring jazz music. Days when a loaf of bread cost a dime and a pound of flour sold for less. Mary Pickford, Al Jolson, Charlie Chaplin, and Rudolph Valentino ruled the screen while George Gershwin stirred American audiences with his orchestral works, especially *Rhapsody in Blue* and *An American in Paris*. Favorite sports heroes were boxer Jack Dempsey and home-run hitter Babe Ruth.

But they were also days punctuated by the rattle of Thompson submachine guns, better known as "Tommy guns," when more than five hundred gangland slayings occurred throughout the country as underworld Mobs fought for control of the liquor traffic. And nowhere in the nation was this more evident than in metropolitan Chicago.

Saint Valentine's Day Massacre

Conflict between the two most powerful criminal gangs in Chicago reached its high water mark on the morning of Thursday, February 14, 1929. Al Capone led the South Side Italian gang and "Bugs" Moran the North Side Irish/German gang. Seven members of the latter gang were lined up facing the back wall of a garage of the SMC Cartage Company and shot in a volley of some six dozen machine gun bullets and two shotgun blasts. The event was carefully planned and carried out by Capone's men, and they exalted in the success of the operation. Yet, unbeknownst to them at the time, it would mark the beginning of the end for the North Side gang and a softening of Capone's control because of stepped-up public outcry and reinforced police intervention.

But what bearing does the above background have on the Brown's Chicken case seventy years later—murders that were unrelated to gangs? It provides both a strange irony and contrast. The number of victims was the same: seven. The location was the same: the greater Chicago area, which has carried the dubious distinction of "the crime capital of America." The contrast rests in the victims of the massacre.

In the 1920s, the community's attitude toward crime was essentially blasé. Until the Saint Valentine's Day incident, most crime there—*even murder*—was met by little more than a yawn. But the massacre was the beginning of the end for murder sprees. Given the public outrage, the reign of even the glorified Al Capone came to an end. Once he was subdued in prison, a relative calm enveloped Chicago—that is, until 1993.

OVERVIEW OF THE CRIME

Palatine, Illinois—January 8, 1993

On a snowy night, Brown's Chicken & Pasta restaurant began closing shortly after 9:00 p.m. in Palatine, a quiet town of forty-two thousand inhabitants. This suburb of Chicago is located on the corner of Northwest Highway and Smith Street, not far from O'Hare Airport. Owners Richard and Lynn Ehlenfeldt had purchased the business the previous year from Frank Portillo, a founder of the 115-restaurant chain, who had proudly added family-style pasta to its menu in order to compete with the giant KFC franchise. The Ehlenfeldts would be two of the seven killed in the bloodiest crime in suburban Chicago history, along with five employees.

The victims were:

- Owner Richard E. Ehlenfeldt, age fifty. Born and raised in Columbus, Wisconsin, Richard studied to become a Methodist minister at one time but was lured into Democratic politics. He worked in the presidential campaigns of George McGovern, Hubert Humphrey, Robert Kennedy, and Jimmy Carter. He also served as Wisconsin's assistant secretary of state.

- Lynn, his forty-nine-year-old wife and co-owner, who also grew up in Wisconsin. After their marriage, she became an avid child-rights advocate, devoting herself to people with developmental disabilities, the hungry, and the homeless.

At the time of their deaths, the Ehlenfeldts had been married for twenty-five years and had three daughters, Jennifer, Dana, and Joy. They purchased the restaurant in 1992, less than a year before the massacre, pouring their life savings into the franchise.

- Guadalupe Maldonado, forty-seven, was a resident of Palatine and worked a shift from 1 p.m. to 9 p.m. as the restaurant's cook. He; his wife, Beatriz; and their thirteen-year-old son, Juan Pablo, were Mexican immigrants who moved to the United States in 1981. Eventually the couple had two more sons, Javier and Salvador. The hardworking father took on different jobs to support his family, usually as a cook.
- Thomas Mennes, thirty-two, was a native of Palatine and a high school dropout. A bachelor and one of twins, he had considerable experience in various food service jobs. Friends said he was a loner, yet friendly and easygoing.
- Marcus Nellsen, also from Palatine, was thirty-one. He was a US Navy veteran who hoped to become Brown's manager. In 1992 he lost his job at a manufacturing plant when it closed. Divorced, he lived for eighteen months in a YMCA before moving in with his girlfriend, Joy. They planned on marrying.
- Sixteen-year-old Michael Castro was a Palatine High School student, the youngest of four children, and a second-generation Filipino American. He worked part-time at Brown's and enjoyed music, dancing, radio-controlled cars, and driving his white Nissan pickup truck.
- Rico Solis, seventeen, and was very close friends with Castro; the two even dressed alike. He was the youngest of three children and emigrated with his mother to the United States in 1992. Ear-

lier, his father had been stabbed to death in the Philippines. Solis drove a 1984 red Dodge Charger and was saving money to buy a newer car.[1]

According to court documents, selected testimony, and a detailed videotape of the crime scene in the immediate hours after the murders, the following represents a likely forty-minute scenario. It is reinforced by what prosecutors claimed were eventual confessions from two men, both just out of high school at the time of the killings.

A few minutes after 9 p.m., the two young men entered Brown's side door. They chose closing time because they figured there would be fewer people inside. One of them, eighteen-year-old Juan Luna, had once worked at the restaurant and knew its layout; he was also aware that it had no burglar alarm system. The other was James Degorski, age twenty. The court documents indicated that the two men liked to "get high" and listen to heavy metal music, and often "abused and tortured animals." On this January night, the prosecutors claimed, the young men had planned to "do something big." It was alleged that their initial intent was to commit a robbery, but this did not jibe with their actions at the scene: Their pockets were filled with bullets, and they wedged the back door shut so no one could escape. In any event, after meeting resistance from the restaurant's employees, they went on their unimaginable killing spree.

Luna first ordered a four-piece chicken meal and Degorski chided him for it. Luna apparently did this as a means of staying in the restaurant until all other customers had left. After calmly eating part of the chicken dinner, he dumped the remains into a trash can, walked toward the counter, and heard Degorski say, "O.K., let's do it."[2]

Luna was following one worker toward the back of the restaurant when he heard a gunshot near the front counter. He turned and saw that Degorski had shot at an employee who attempted to jump over the counter.

The men rounded up the male employees and herded them into a walk-in cooler and a walk-in freezer. Luna next had Lynn Ehlenfeldt open the safe and then ordered her into the freezer. When she resisted, he slit her throat with a hunting knife. The two men then used Degorski's .38 caliber pistol to shoot the victims, firing at least twenty rounds between them.

At 3:11 a.m., police found two bodies in the west-side cooler—those of Richard Ehlenfeldt and Mennes—and the other five bodies piled on top of each other in the east-side freezer. The victims had bullet holes in the back of the head, leading authorities to believe it was an execution-style massacre, with the victims forced to kneel before being shot. The youngest victims, Castro and Solis, were shot more than once—Castro was shot six times. In addition, Castro was stabbed in the abdomen after he died. This suggested that Castro and Solis had tried to fend off their attackers.

When it was over, Degorski mopped up most of the blood. At 9:48 p.m. (as indicated by the reading on an electric clock inside the restaurant), Luna threw the circuit breaker to turn off the lights. The two men then walked out of the restaurant with approximately $1,800 from the safe.

Later, investigators found bullets in cardboard boxes and jars of gravy, and under soda machines. A total of about twenty bullets were recovered from the victims' bodies and the crime scene.

There was at least a five-hour delay in the discovery of the bodies, a fact that would later contribute to a condemnation of the Palatine police and other law enforcement officials. In the early morning hours of the next day, January 9, several of the victims' family members arrived at the restaurant looking for their relatives but were stopped by policemen in the parking lot. Pedro Maldonado, Guadalupe's brother, and Emmanuel Castro, Michael's father, claimed the officers were not aware of the crime and did not bother to look inside the building at the time. There was later a general feeling among many—not only concerned family members—that precious time had been wasted, that perhaps some lives could have been saved. Another lapse cited was that the police failed to canvass the area immediately. If they had, they would have discovered that a nearby twenty-four-hour gas station had a security video camera in operation that might have captured the murderers on tape before or after their crime. But existence of the camera did not come to light until two weeks later; by then the tape from the night in question had been erased and reused.[3]

The Two Suspects

Juan Luna and James Degorski had been classmates at Palatine's William Fremd High School at the time of the 1993 tragedy. Unlike Degorski, Luna had no criminal record except for an isolated bounced check episode years later, in 1999. His parents, Juan Sr. and Alicia, said that, like nearly everyone in the Chicago area, the family had heard about the murders when they occurred but never suspected the highly publicized crime would touch their lives. The couple stated they could not accept what the Palatine police had said about their son—that he was a person "without a soul." They characterized him as a compassionate, religious man who had never given his family any cause for concern. "Juan would go to church with his family, he would pray and ask forgiveness. That's why it hurts when they said he did those things, because I know my son," his mother said.[4]

In high school, he enrolled in the work-study program with Degorski and also with Eileen Bakalla, who would later play a key role in the arrests and at Luna's trial.

In 1994, a year after the homicides, Luna married a Mexican woman named Imelda, and they settled into an apartment in suburban northwest Chicago. Three years later, their son, Brian, was born.

Degorski, on the other hand, had crossed paths with the police on numerous occasions. During the three years prior to the murders, he was charged with auto theft, burglary, battery, and unlawful restraint. After 1993 he was arrested for marijuana possession, driving under the influence of alcohol, and several traffic violations. As numerous as the charges were, they paled in comparison to the number of times he moved—from Illinois to Arizona and back—and the number of jobs he held in different areas, including home remodeling, golf course maintenance, office cleaning, and window shutter installation, among others.

As indicated above, both men had an early history of drug use and exhibited bizarre behavior, including the torture of small animals. Some police sources believed that on that terrible winter night, they were looking for a person to kill—any person. But none could fathom why it turned out to be seven; why, in the span of forty-four minutes, two young men became mass murderers.

A year after the crime, it became a cold case. And it took nine more years for clues to be discovered that would eventually lead to arrests and indictments.

1993 to Early 2002

Within minutes of the discovery of the bodies, investigators from the Cook County Sheriff's Department and the Northern Illinois Police Crime Laboratory swung into action. The restaurant and its parking lot were secured. Even police detectives were banned from the area until evidence gathering had been completed. Those allowed inside the building were required to wear disposable gloves and foot protectors. Forensic technicians dusted for fingerprints, measured blood spatter, took swabs, and photographed bodies. They retrieved nearly a hundred fingerprints, along with hairs, fibers, blood, and bullets. All business records were confiscated. Investigators spotted a bloody mop resting near the east door and theorized that the killers had used it to clean the scene of blood. Bloody prints dotted the door frame of the freezer. A bullet hole was discovered in the ceiling. The safe had a key in its lock. No spent shell casings were found. Money was discovered in the sock of one victim and the wallet of another. Still another victim's credit card was located behind some boxes. An empty drinking cup rested on the counter. One of the investigators recovered a receipt from the cash register. It described the last order placed the night before: four pieces of chicken, rolls, and a drink. The time posted at the top of the slip was 21:07.

Notably, the lead forensic scientist from the northern Illinois lab, Jane Homeyer, twenty-nine, was among those scouring the restaurant.

She was to assume a pivotal role in the investigation and later as a witness in Juan Luna's trial. Her reputation was that of an exceptional scientist; she had begun her career working on forgeries and handwriting analysis. She later became executive director of the Highland Park crime lab and, later still, director of the forensic training unit at the FBI Academy in Quantico, Virginia.

Rummaging through several garbage containers, Homeyer observed that all but one were empty. In the plastic liner bag of that single container, she found the bones and gristle of a chicken meal and a paper napkin. She was not sure if such a finding would ever be of any evidentiary value, but gathered up the meal anyway and ensured that it was frozen so it could be analyzed at a future date. Improved bite-mark technology and the possible extraction of DNA from dried saliva on the chicken bones were foremost in her mind. In those days, DNA analysis was in its relative infancy, but Homeyer knew that such testing was becoming more sophisticated at a rapid pace.

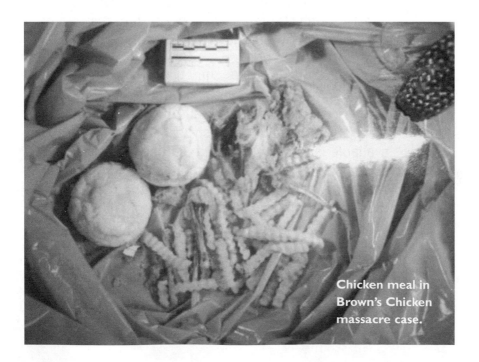

Chicken meal in Brown's Chicken massacre case.

In **Henry Lee's Crime Scene Handbook,** Timothy Palmbach, Marilyn Miller, and I wrote the following, much of which is relevant to this case:

- In the earlier parts of last century criminal investigations were dependent on the ability of law enforcement officials to obtain information from witnesses and suspects, or on the use of informants or undercover operations. If interviews or interrogations failed to provide the needed investigative information, or no informants were available, often the cases remained unsolved.
- Contemporary law enforcement has greatly expanded its ability to solve crimes by the adoption of techniques and procedures that recognize the importance of the combined powers of crime scenes, physical evidence, records, and witnesses in successful criminal investigations. Today's crimes are most often solved by a system that focuses on teamwork, advanced investigative skills, and the ability to process a crime scene properly; that is, recognizing, collecting, and preserving all relevant physical evidence and information.
- However, numerous routine and high-profile cases have demonstrated the harsh reality that, despite available current crime scene technologies and specialized personnel, the effectiveness of crime scene functions [is] only as good as the management system that supports those functions.
- For centuries, crimes have been solved traditionally through interrogation in order to generate leads for investigators. However, since the early 1970s many court decisions have severely constrained police and fire investigators in their use of traditional interrogation techniques. With new

developments in crime scene technology the investigator has realized that the crime scene contains a tremendous amount of information. This information can often link a suspect to a crime scene, prove or disprove an alibi, or develop investigative leads. Information can be in oral form, written statements or documents, or in the form of pattern evidence. Information can be derived from individuals at the scene, forensic evidence located [at] or remarked absent from the scene, or pattern evidence located within the scene. The sooner the information can be recognized, analyzed, collected, and preserved, the better chance that the case will be solved.

- Many cases have been ultimately solved not by a lengthy scientific analysis, but rather by the properly documented, seemingly insignificant detail located or observed at the crime scene. Quality documentation includes photographs, videotaping, preparation of sketch maps, and other forms of written or audio/visual recording formats.
- Information located at a scene comes in different forms requiring different methods to properly recognize, collect, and preserve such information. Some of the information . . . is in the form of physical evidence. Physical evidence is what we generally perceive to be forensic evidence, such as the murder weapon or bullet casing. However, in any given case any particular object may prove to be the crucial piece of physical evidence [needed] to solve the case.[5]

In this case, albeit after many years, the chicken bones found and preserved by Jane Homeyer turned out to be the crucial piece of evidence. It seemed destined to help solve a prolonged story, one straight out of a Sherlock Holmes mystery. Its importance cannot be overemphasized for there were no known witnesses. Years later, however, more information would suddenly hatch from the most unlikely sources—from two informants and from the two suspects themselves.

Authorities were baffled from the start. They were not certain of the number of guns used or even of the number of killers involved. Within three days, Palatine police chief Jerry Bratcher did the correct thing in forming the Palatine Task Force, seventy-five strong, consisting of local and state police together with FBI personnel. But it wasn't long before critics became highly vocal in claiming a lack of progress in the overall investigation, and this criticism became increasingly vitriolic as time passed. They charged that the Palatine police were not up to the task, that the crime lab was incompetent, and that potentially valuable tips were being ignored.

In the many months ahead, little meaningful progress was made and the case became very cold. These were times filled with false leads, phony confessions, and bitter confrontations among politicians, community and business leaders, the media, and law enforcement representatives. Meanwhile, the city of Palatine had changed dramatically because memories of that bloody night continued to haunt the northwest suburb.

"Palatine is not a town that gets hysterical about things, but this hit at our heart," said a friend of Michael Castro, one of the victims.

Another longtime resident said, "Before the killings, Palatine was a place where doors went unlocked and personal safety was taken for granted."

Still another stated, "Everybody knew everybody. You watched out for your neighbor's kids. Every kid had ten moms on the block."

And in what appeared to become the dominant theme of the change, a seasoned retiree commented, "Everyone started looking at everyone. They didn't know if they trusted anybody."[6]

In short, the public was both up in arms and scared. And the situation worsened as the months became years—nine years, in fact. At the beginning of this lengthy period, the task force grew to 120 members, but within two years it was scaled down to seven full-time investigators. It was around this time that Frank Portillo, owner and chief executive officer of Brown's Chicken & Pasta, asked the Chicago Crime Commission (CCC) and the Better Government Association (BGA) to examine the task force's handling of the investigation.

On January 28, 1994, I was contacted by Bratcher and Assistant District Attorney Patrick W. O'Brien to assist the task force by examining the physical evidence and conducting a crime scene reconstruction.

I flew to Chicago, where several detectives met me at the airport and drove me to police headquarters. After a detailed briefing by some task force members, I met with Bratcher, the rest of the task force members, the district attorney's investigators, and FBI and laboratory personnel. I spent the rest of the day at the Brown's Chicken restaurant to re-create the original crime scene and establish a possible sequence of events. Then, well into the night, I studied hundreds of photographs and reviewed thousands of pages of reports and statements.

The next day I examined each piece of physical evidence: bullets, the victims' clothing, bottles, cans, fibers, blood, hairs, and, of course, the liner of the garbage can (which particularly caught my attention). It was extremely clean and contained only a small amount of garbage. It appeared that only a chicken wing had been eaten. In checking the cash register receipts, we found that the last meal, sold at 9:07 p.m., contained four pieces of chicken. (See report below.)

I worked with the task force through that night, examining each item of physical evidence and focusing on the chicken pieces. These had been stored in a freezer in the Northern Illinois Crime Lab. (This facility was the only regional crime lab in northern Illinois at the time. The Chicago city lab was under the jurisdiction of the Chicago City Police. Later, both labs merged into the state forensic lab system, located in Springfield.)

On the third day I met with Bratcher and the rest of the investigators in order to brief them on my findings and conclusions. I first indicated that the task force had done an excellent job and that, had any luck been on its side, there might have been a major breakthrough. I also indicated that DNA should be extracted from the chicken wing, pointing out that the wing was most likely eaten by a suspect and that his chewing action would have resulted in the transfer of his saliva to the bone. Such saliva would contain cheek cells, which in turn would contain his nuclear DNA. Once DNA results were obtained, we could compare them with those from any suspects or we could search the DNA data bank and possibly have a DNA "hit"—all of which would go a long way in solving the case.

Subsequently, I issued the following report to Bratcher and the task force on January 28, 1994:

CONNECTICUT STATE FORENSIC LABORATORY
RECONSTRUCTION REPORT
INTRODUCTION:

On January 9, 1993, seven bodies were found in the cooler areas of the Brown's Chicken Restaurant at 168 W. Northwest Highway, Palatine, IL. On January 28, 1994, Dr. Henry Lee of the Connecticut State Police Forensic Science Laboratory was contacted by Chief Jerry Bratcher of the Palatine Police Department and Attorney Patrick W. O'Brien, Special Prosecutor in Cook County, Illinois to review evidence and to assist in the case investigation. From February 10 through 15, 1994, Dr. Lee met the investigative team, visited the crime scene, reviewed documents and photographs, and reexamined several pieces of physical evidence. After reviewing documents and photographs, and examining physical evidence, the following observations were made.

1. The homicide scene was located at Brown's Chicken Restaurant, 168 W. Northwest Highway, Palatine, Illinois. All seven victims were shot and died as a result of multiple gunshot wounds. In addition, two of the victims also had knife wounds.

2. A large amount of cash receipts for the day was missing from the restaurant. The scene was consistent with a robbery-homicide type of case.

3. Firearm, footwear imprint, fingerprint and a variety of other physical evidence were collected from this restaurant by detectives of the Palatine Police Department and forensic scientists from the Northern Illinois Crime Laboratory. This evidence was submitted to the Northern Illinois Crime Laboratory for analysis.

4. Police evidence submission lists indicate that approximately 22 bullet/bullet fragments were submitted for examination. These bullet/bullet fragments were examined microscopically. Results indicate that trace evidence was observed on some of the items.

5. The exact number of individual latent prints and palm prints developed during the examinations was not determined. All the latent prints developed at the scene and on items of evidence seized from the scene were examined by Latent Print Examiners of the Northern Illinois Crime Laboratory.

6. The exact number of individual footwear imprints developed during the examination was not determined. All the footwear imprints were examined by examiners of the Northern Illinois Crime Laboratory.

7. One of the items of physical evidence was collected from a garbage can in the west side of the restaurant. This item consisted of a chicken meal from the restaurant, labeled as "0093–157–9, 01/8/93–12/04/93." This item was stored in a freezer at Northern Illinois Crime Laboratory.

8. This item was taken out of the freezer and examined macroscopically and microscopically by Dr. Lee at the Serology Section of the Northern Illinois Crime Laboratory. The following items were found in the evidence:

(1) Thirty seven (37) strips of French fries
(2) Two (2) intact biscuits
(3) One (1) intact chicken leg
(4) One (1) intact chicken breast
(5) One (1) portion of chicken
(6) One (1) portion of chicken wing
(7) Five (5) pieces of bone remains
(8) Paper napkins, plates, box, stirrer, cups and a variety of other materials.

9. The five (5) small pieces of chicken bone appeared to be the remains of a portion of a chicken meal which was eaten by an individual or individuals.

10. The crime scene documentation, location and condition of the chicken meal, sales receipts of the last meal, and time that this last chicken meal was sold, all indicate that the physical evidence found on this chicken meal is a very important [lead] toward linking a suspect to this case.

These observations and conclusions are based on a review of the submitted crime scene documentation, and the examination of the previously described items [of] physical evidence. This conclusion may [be] subject to change and/or modification based on submission of any new materials or information.[7]

On April 17, 1996, it was announced that an independent Blue Ribbon Panel had been formed "to review and provide recommendations concerning the handling of murder investigations like the 1993 Brown's Chicken homicides." The announcement stated that members "were selected for their expertise in law enforcement, legal education and the public interest, and [the panel] is composed of former high-level federal, state and city law enforcement investigators, officials, prosecutors and academic experts."[8]

The presence and role of these advisory/watchdog groups seemed confounding to some, if only in terms of their numbers. Stated another way, it was difficult to keep them straight. And while some critics hailed the work of each one of them, others claimed the Chicago area was "over-paneled."

The Chicago Crime Commission and the Better Government Association, both ongoing bodies, had arisen during the era of Al Capone in response to his ascent to power as well as increasing instances of political corruption and other government transgressions. On the other hand, the task force, assembled on an ad hoc basis, was formed shortly after the Brown's Chicken massacre. And finally, the BGA and CCC formed the independent Blue Ribbon Panel. Its avowed purpose was "not to solve the crime but to answer some basic questions about whether appropriate resources were deployed in a manner consistent with the professional law enforcement standards which the community has a right to expect."[9]

Many of the panel's determinations received widespread public support. It announced, for example, that although the Palatine Police Department was sincere in its desire to solve the crime, it was inexperienced in major homicide investigations. Yet after the task force was assembled, Palatine officers, rather than more experienced officers who then became available, still remained in key positions of responsibility on the task force. The panel went on to say that the less experienced officers were overwhelmed by the magnitude of the case and failed effectively to secure the crime scene, to canvass the surrounding area, to coordinate investigative personnel—especially in utilizing those who were more experienced than they were in homicide investigations, to integrate the variety of resources (e.g., various computer database and analysis capabilities) that were available from the wide range of law enforcement agencies comprising the task force, and to open basic lines of communication between the command and rank and file within the task force. This inexperience, they said, contributed not only to a delayed discovery of the crime scene, but it also wasted three days of investigative efforts pursuing one lead, subsequently proven false, while ignoring all other investigative avenues.

With respect to the state's attorney's office, the panel stated the office departed from its traditional role of allowing the police to solve the crime, instead insinuating itself into a murder investigation and eventually emerging as a leader of the task force. This in turn resulted in having state's attorney's investigative personnel who were inexperienced in major homicide investigations placed into key tactical command positions. Such an approach contributed to a failure to share critical investigative information among task force investigators, bungling in the surveillance of a prime suspect, internal disputes that resulted in the inappropriate release of a prime suspect, feuding among experienced investigators from the various agencies over the handling of a crucial lead, a continuing lack of confidence in the leadership by many task force members, and finally, the disintegration of the task force.

The panel asserted that the above command mistakes led quickly to a defensive posture with the media and the public. They contended that this posture then led to placing more emphasis on creating a positive PR "spin" rather than forming an effective law enforcement team, and some of that spin was often contradicted by the facts available to the task force.

With all of the above in mind, it came as no surprise that the Blue Ribbon Panel's ultimate and firm recommendation was: "The Village Trustees and the Mayor of Palatine should have then, now and in the future provide oversight to the police department's conduct and performance to ensure they have sufficient means necessary to conduct a major homicide investigation."[10]

Adding to these scathing remarks, *Police Chief* magazine, a national publication, observed, "Certainly the traditional safeguarding of turf is a problem in many jurisdictions. Some Chiefs feel threatened by the suggestion that they are unable to successfully investigate a homicide without the assistance of outside experts. Unfortunately, they may be protecting their own egos at the victim's expense as the murder goes unsolved."[11]

But it wasn't just the task force that had been receiving bad publicity. The Brown's Chicken massacre had been the top story of the television and print media on practically a daily basis. This combined with the fact that the killer or killers had still not been caught led frightened customers to shy away from Frank Portillo's restaurants.

"For those first few weeks, actually for most of that first year, it seemed to me that we were on the television news morning, afternoon, and night," he later said.[12]

Even his employees, fearing the murders were the work of a serial killer, resigned en masse. By the end of 1993, sales had dwindled by 20 percent. And within the next year, Emmanuel Castro, the father of one of the victims, filed a lawsuit against the Brown's chain. A short time later, Rico Solis's family did the same thing.

"I was very hurt by that," Portillo stated, "and at that time I went to Bratcher to ask him for just enough information to cover myself against the lawsuits." Portillo later recalled, "He said no, that it was an ongoing investigation. I was not happy, but by then my relationship with the police was fizzling anyway. I was becoming a pretty vocal critic of the police.... But what they didn't understand was that I wasn't criticizing the department so much as the system. There's something wrong with the system, where small-town police who don't have experience have jurisdiction over more experienced homicide detectives. I think they were working as hard as they could. They wanted to solve this. They just weren't qualified. Look at it this way: I'm president of fifty-eight restaurants. McDonald's has twenty-seven billion or something. So do they come to me and say, 'Hey, you want to be president of our corporation?' I could work seven days a week, but I still wouldn't be qualified. It's the same thing with a small town."[13]

For his part, Bratcher tried to remain above the fray—maintaining a professional attitude—but it was common knowledge that he was fuming over the various reports and negative opinions. He adamantly said the police and task force would not cooperate in any way, especially with handing over internal reports and allowing interviews with task force members. "These are people of integrity, so I'm not going to blast them," he said. "I don't know the mission that's been developed for them, but it's more than a little puzzling to me why [the various critics] would accept this if they knew the whole story."[14]

A year after that statement, in 1997, with four years of no progress, the BGA issued an even more blistering report criticizing the handling of the case. It contended that the crime scene had been compromised, the police crime lab was a disaster, and that Bratcher was self-serving. (I have known the chief for many years—even before the Brown's Chicken massacre—and can attest to the fact that he is an excellent chief and a good person. But his reputation was hurt by this difficult case.)

It didn't stop there, however. Three years later—seven years after the massacre—yet another report captured the headlines. Its title was simple enough: "Without Merit"—referring to the BGA report. A panel of experts assembled by the Illinois State Crime Commission (ISCC) had dissected the BGA report and concluded that "[t]he Palatine Police Department and Brown's Chicken Task Force and its members acted professionally, followed all leads and conducted the investigation thoroughly. In short, the Better Government Association's conclusions are not based upon fact."[15]

The attorney who led the team of experts stated publicly, "There's no way this investigation was botched. We looked behind the criticism and we found that the BGA report—95 percent of it—was baseless. We found the Palatine Police Department and the other law enforcement agencies worked properly; they had harmony. A superb investigative [and] follow-through job. We have no criticism. Unfortunately, some crimes never get solved."[16]

The ISCC report took exception to most of the BGA's assertions. To cite a few examples, it stated that the BGA's description of the crime scene was incorrect. It indicated that there was no "parade" in the restaurant, that the only personnel allowed inside were employees of the medical examiner's office, the lead investigators, and crime scene technicians—and all were required to wear protective clothing, including gloves and booties over their shoes. The report went on to say that all the victims had been fingerprinted, that complete canvassing of the area had taken place, and that the crime lab had performed its duties in a professional and proper fashion. It noted that at the end of the first year of the investigation, the task force had brought in several investigators to conduct a "cold case review." These investigators included Kirk Mellecker, a very experienced retired Los Angeles homicide detective and "Dr. Henry Lee, [Connecticut's chief forensic scientist made famous in many high-profile case investigations. They] had concurred with the Task Force's theory of the case."[17] Mellecker "determined that a complete and thorough job was done investigating suspects, performing investigative tasks, preserving evidence and utilizing 'ALL' tools available."[18]

And so it went for nine emotional years: the finger-pointing and infighting among the police, other law enforcement agencies, the politicians, the owner of the Brown's chain, the business establishment, the community at large, and some of the victims' family members. Before it was over, there were reports on panels, panels on reports, reports on reports, and panels on panels.

Meanwhile, the killers remained at large.

THE BIG BREAK

A phone conversation on March 25, 2002, brought revelations that would dramatically change the complexion of the case. Anne Lockett, twenty-six, made contact with an on-again, off-again friend from high school. This friend would prove pivotal to the case, though she has refused to reveal her name to this day. At the time, Lockett was sharing an apartment with her boyfriend in Charleston, a tiny town two hundred miles southwest of Chicago. She was taking psychology classes and was gainfully employed, working with developmentally disabled adults.

As later recounted by the "friend," Lockett had called her to ask for a favor: Would she be willing to forward an anonymous letter to the police? When pressed, Lockett grudgingly stated that the letter would deal with a crime and that it could not be postmarked from Charleston. But the friend said she wouldn't cooperate unless she was given more details. Eventually, Lockett revealed that she had been hiding from Jim Degorski and Juan Luna. The friend remembered them both as part of a high school group that hung out at a certain pizza joint. She also recalled that Lockett and Degorski had been romantically involved for about two years, frequently smoking marijuana together, and that he was both physically and emotionally abusive to her. Characterized as controlling, he even insisted Lockett abandon her previous circle of friends. In contrast, the friend's memory of Luna was vague, but she was aware of a friendship between him and Degorski.

When queried about the reason for her wanting to hide from them, Lockett opened up, and it soon became clear why she had never come forward, why she had chosen instead to deal with a secret torment for so many years. She presented a step-by-step account of what she had probably buried in a troubled mind—and a terrified soul.

Degorski, she said, had phoned her on the night of January 9, 1993—a day after the massacre—and asked her to check the television stations. The call was made to Forest Hospital where Lockett was a patient, apparently for depression. She was seventeen at the time and the prevailing rumor, although not substantiated, was that she had just gone through her fifth suicide attempt.

"Watch the news," he said. "I did something."[19] Lockett complied and discovered that seven people had been murdered in a Brown's restaurant and that there were no leads regarding the perpetrator or perpetrators. Shortly thereafter, she, Degorski, and Luna sat together in Degorski's bedroom, where the two men described how they had killed the seven victims. Their conversation lasted a long time, Luna speaking in an animated fashion. Degorski was more measured, almost businesslike, and Lockett felt that he was the leader of the two men.

What follows is a condensed version of what she learned and told her friend—and later admitted to the police.

Luna said he had wanted to kill someone; Degorski said he would help. They chose the Brown's restaurant because Luna had once worked there, knew the layout, and also knew there was no security system in place. They dressed in old clothes and took many bullets with them. Armed with Degorski's snub-nosed .38 caliber handgun, they drove Luna's Ford Tempo to a parking lot near the restaurant and then walked in a deliberately erratic way in an effort to disguise their gaits and shoeprints in the snow. (In fact, on the way back, they stepped in their own shoeprints.) They inserted a wedge in the restaurant's back door so that no one could slip out. They entered at closing time and Luna ordered a chicken dinner. This angered Degorski, because the chicken was greasy and he said that fingerprints might become more obvious. Luna ate some of the chicken; they both put on gloves and then brandished the gun. A scuffle ensued with one of the employees. Another one raced to the back door; unable to open it, he ran to the front, leaped over the counter, and was shot, presumably by Degorski. The two assailants then herded the victims into the cooler and freezer. In the process, Lynn Ehlenfeldt angered Luna, so he called her a bitch and proceeded to cut her throat. During the shooting spree that followed, one of the victims vomited french fries. Assured that all seven were dead (one of the killers even jabbed at one with a mop in order to be certain), they grabbed the money in the safe, left in a hurry, and tossed the gun in the Fox River.

A few days later, Luna called Degorski's house. Lockett was there. Luna informed them that since he had once been an employee at Brown's, the task force wanted to question him. Both Luna and Lockett went to the police station, and Luna's interview lasted less than thirty minutes. He told Lockett the interview seemed routine but they had photographed him.

Lockett said that neither man spoke to her again about the massacre—that the last reference to it was when Degorski had issued a sharp warning: "If you ever tell anyone about this, I will kill you."[20]

THE ARRESTS

Minutes after she hung up the phone, the stunned and agitated friend put in a call to a police officer she had befriended years before. Moments earlier, Lockett had given her permission to do so. The officer was not on duty at the time, but, after a series of delays and with the friend's nervousness at a fever pitch, contact was finally made later that night. The officer, intrigued but cautious, indicated that Palatine detective sergeant Bill King would call her back. Members of the Palatine police force had been done in too often by false leads and bogus suspects, and had become leery of tips because none had ever panned out. As later recalled by the friend, "They ... had about 15,000 tips about this thing, but nothing had ever come of [them]." Speaking of King, she added, "He had received hundreds of phone calls about it, and I'm sure he [initially] thought this was just another tip that would lead to nothing."[21]

The friend, however, sensed that King was encouraged. This time the detective, the only one remaining on the case from the start, seemed determined to follow through on Lockett's revelation to her friend. He seized information as if starved for it, checking and double-checking, asking question after question. This time was, in fact, totally different. Lockett had disclosed something that had never before been released to the media: that one of the victims had vomited french fries during the shootings. It was information that only the real killers could know.

The friend heard nothing from the police for days, during which time she agonized over two things: (1) the possibility that if the men were prosecuted, she might be called as a witness at their trial; and (2) the fear of being killed herself. She and her roommate made doubly sure that their doors and windows were kept locked.

Two weeks after she spoke with King, Palatine's new police chief, John Koziol, appeared at her apartment. He was accompanied by Cook County sheriff's police commander John Robertson and assistant Cook County state's attorney Scott Cassidy. They questioned her for hours. Later she recollected, "These guys were so on the ball. They went over every single nitty, gritty thing. They wanted to get in their car and drive to see Anne [Lockett] right then."[22] The friend telephoned Lockett, but there was no answer.

The police subsequently reviewed the investigative report of Luna's interview with the task force in 1993. He had claimed that on the night of the killings, he was with a high school friend named Eileen Bakalla. The report indicated that the police had spoken with her immediately afterward and she had confirmed what Luna had said.

Now it was time for authorities to interrogate her again. She stated that on January 8, 1993—the night of the murders—she was working at Jake's Pizza when she received a call from Degorski. He asked her to meet him in the parking lot of a nearby grocery store. "We did something big," he said. When she arrived, both Degorski and Luna were in Luna's car. She recalled seeing latex gloves on the car's console and noted that Luna held a canvas bag. They decided to drive to her roommate's townhouse in Elgin, a twenty-minute ride southwest of Palatine. On the way, they told her they had robbed the Brown's Chicken restaurant. (She did not indicate a clear-cut reaction to the news.) At the townhouse, the men emptied the canvas bag of money, gave Bakalla fifty dollars, and split the rest between them. She said they then smoked pot until dawn.

Armed with Lockett's and Bakalla's disclosures—each story supporting the other—the police believed they had enough to proceed to the next step. They located Luna at a gas station in Carpentersville, northwest of Chicago, and Degorski in Indianapolis. Each was asked permission to have the inside of his cheek swabbed for DNA—providing a so-called buccal smear. Both willingly consented; Luna's sample was obtained at his home, Degorski's at a Palatine lab. Authorities were amazed that neither man resisted having the procedure performed.

Of this, one investigator commented, "It was easy for Luna—he had worked at Brown's and it didn't seem unusual that this was being done. For Degorski, I don't know. Maybe he thought that if he refused, he would look guilty. And if he had, we would have gotten a court order."[23]

On May 8, the result of the DNA analysis indicated that Luna's matched the DNA profile from the partially eaten chicken meal that had been dumped into one of the garbage containers at the crime scene and kept frozen for years. The technicians cited a chance of one in more than a trillion that the match could be wrong. Both men were placed under twenty-four-hour surveillance.

Three days later, investigators, having methodically plotted their next course of action, returned to Anne Lockett for additional help. Their scheme was to have her phone Degorski, state that the police had begun asking her questions about the murders, and inquire about what she should say. Eventually, after Lockett repeated her story under oath before a Cook County grand jury, a court order was obtained allowing her phone to be tapped during a call to Degorski. He neither admitted nor denied taking part in the crime, but such a stance did little to convince the police of his innocence.

Thus, on Thursday, May 16, 2002, Juan Luna and James Degorski were arrested and charged with seven counts of first-degree murder while committing a robbery. After hours of questioning, Luna agreed to give a videotaped statement to assistant state's attorney Darren O'Brien and investigator Brian Killacky. In the tape, Luna spoke in monotone and outlined what had transpired on that fateful 1993 night.

"I figured it would be simple," Luna said softly. His role, he stated, was to ensure that no one ran out the doors, while Degorski was to act as the "aggressive one."

"With everything going all wild and crazy . . . I guess I got caught up in the moment." After the victims were forced into the freezer, Luna claimed, Degorski told him to shoot into it. "I wasn't really aiming for anybody to get shot or anything like that, just to scare them because I didn't want to hurt anybody," he said. "They were yelling, 'Don't shoot us, please don't shoot us.' Their hands were shaking." Luna then lowered his voice further and concluded with, "I feel so sad and I'm so sorry. . . . If I could do this all again, there's no way in hell I'd do this at all."[24]

When asked to comment on the videotape, University of San Francisco law professor Richard Leo said defense lawyers would have diffi-

culty getting a jury to believe that someone would have falsely confessed to a multiple murder. Leo, an expert in police interrogation and
confessions, said, "I think there's no worse evidence to have against you
other than a videotape that catches you in the act or a DNA test." He
added that defense lawyers nonetheless often claim coercion when
there is a confession.[25]

Prosecutors contended that there was never any evidence that Luna
was abused or misled. But Luna countered that police slapped and
punched him to get him to talk and promised he could leave if he
admitted his involvement. He alleged that investigators fed him details,
which he repeated for the camera, and that police threatened to deport
his family back to Mexico.

Furthermore, prosecutors were expected to show in court that the
chance of anyone other than Luna being linked to the DNA findings
was 1 in 2.8 trillion. Therefore, the defense would have to work very
hard in trying to get the jury to treat DNA like any other evidence, said
William Thompson, chairman of criminology, law, and society at the
University of California at Irvine.

"It's very effective with jurors," Thompson stated. "DNA is typically treated as the gold standard and is given tremendous credibility
unless the defense can come up with very specific attacks on it."[26]

For their part, defense lawyers were expected to argue that investigators improperly stored the chicken samples, destroyed the original
bags that contained the chicken, and discarded a computer that held
data pertaining to the DNA. "The evidence was commingled with other
evidence. It's our position there would be no clear link linking Juan
Luna's DNA," said one of Luna's attorneys, Clarence Burch.[27]

At a news conference the next day, Friday, Koziol stated, in part:

> [W]e have amassed a formidable case against these cold-blooded
> killers. This evidence includes sworn testimony, court-ordered
> overhears, admissions by the defendants and, most importantly,
> DNA evidence. I want to acknowledge all the fine investigators
> and agencies who have assisted us over the many years in this

case. There were over one hundred and fifty. And to the people charged...you wanted to do something big. I hope you are placed in a cage that you have built through your own inhumanity toward the innocent. I am confident that you will receive the death sentence you so justly deserve. It galls me that these two individuals, who are void of human conscience, took the lives of seven decent, law-abiding Americans. May those seven people, whose faces will be forever etched in our memory, now rest in peace.[28]

At the same conference, Cook County sheriff Michael Sheahan added,

This is a very difficult case and it's been a long time in coming. From day one, the case had had a chilling effect on all of us in law enforcement, on all the people in this community and on all the people in Cook County. The police never gave up. They never...forgot the victims and that's the key here. That's why it's such a great day to see these officers here and all the assistant state's attorneys, the sheriffs, and all the other officers who worked on the case tirelessly for a number of years—over nine years.

He paused and, in a thinly veiled swipe at the BGA, continued, "When you think of this case, there were, I believe—with the other chiefs and for Chief John Koziol—over the years, some unfair criticism. That unfair criticism was about a very difficult case. There were no eyewitnesses. All the victims were dead."[29]

And Cook County state's attorney Dick Devine followed: "When you stop and think of the terrible devastation that was brought to bear on many, many families, on a neighborhood, on the community by that senseless and unforgivable act several years ago, our heart goes out to the families of the victims. . . . We remember the victims, we remember their families and we do make the commitment to all of you that this case will be pursued and we will get justice in the end."[30]

In response to a question from a reporter about the demeanor of Luna and Degorski when they were brought in and during their interrogation, Koziol answered, "Pretty nonchalant. Your typical sociopath type. They never showed any remorse throughout their statements. I cannot explain their motivation for doing this killing. We still cannot give that answer to the families. They never really gave us one. They just did it to do something big.... They are people without a soul."[31]

Burch immediately asked Cook County judge Raymond Myles for a gag order on lawyers and police involved with the investigation. He asserted that comments by public officials since the arrests had been prejudicial to his client and might make it hard to find an impartial jury. "My client has a right to a fair trial, and the veneer of the jury will be selected from this community," Burch said. "What we'd ask is that you tone down the rhetoric so that he can have a fair trial." Among Burch's objections were comments made by Palatine police chief John Koziol at the news conference, such as "They are people without a soul" and "I am confident you will receive the death sentence you so justly deserve."

The defense lawyer continued, "My client has a soul. He's a human being. And that's the ultimate question the jury will decide, whether or not there are any redeeming values that would preclude the death penalty."[32] (To some observers, including the two of us, the attorney's last statement seemed to intimate guilt, since he homed in on a penalty before any verdict had been rendered.)

Joy Sojoodi, one of the Ehlenfeldts' daughters, released a statement. "They had no idea who they took from me and my sisters," she told reporters, fighting back tears. "And I mean, I would like to tell them that I think they're pathetic. And I think my parents would have felt very sorry for them that they were in such a state in their lives like they felt like this was a fun and entertaining thing to do."[33]

"What a waste," said Joy McClain, who had been Marcus Nellsen's fiancée. "Just to get a thrill, they butchered seven people. Those people [the victims] must have been terrified when they realized what was going to happen."[34]

Emmanuel Castro, the father of one of the victims, was unequivocal in his feelings. If given a chance to go to heaven or hell, he said he would choose hell. That way, he reasoned, he could follow Jim Degorski and Juan Luna around for all of eternity and torment them forever. Announcing he was in favor of the death penalty, Castro said, "They killed my son. That's what they deserve. If they're going to the electric chair, I'll put in the plug. I'll pull the switch. If they're given an injection, I'll give the injection. If they're given a firing squad, I'll pull the trigger."[35]

Diane Mennes, the sister-in-law of another victim, said the family was anxious for information. "We're very, very elated and happy, but we're holding [back] because we've had a couple other incidents that they had people not in custody but holding them and then they had to let them go," she said cautiously. "So we're just waiting for the charges now."[36]

Most of the families were perplexed that Lockett and Bakalla went on after the massacre to live apparently normal lives. "They [were] just saving their own butts, that's all," said Mary Jane Crow, Michael Castro's sister.[37]

Continuing to talk with reporters, Diane Mennes offered a different perspective. She told them that if Lockett had come forward before 1998—when DNA testing had become sufficiently sophisticated to isolate a profile from saliva—it might have been a different story. "God works in mysterious ways," she said. "If she would have come forward first, they probably would have thought she was loony tunes. A lot of people were coming forward at the time accusing their [exes]."[38]

Even Frank Portillo, the former owner of Brown's Chicken in Palatine and the man whose harsh words had prompted the BGA report, voiced several opinions: "I know Chief Bratcher wanted to solve the crime just like anyone else. I feel bad I was a critic, and if I could do it all again, I'd take it back. How [Lockett's and Bakalla's] conscience[s] would let them go without talking to the police, how they could live with themselves, I have no idea. What these people did was an act of cruelty."[39]

Myles eventually denied the defense motion for a gag order, stating it was "overly broad and impermissibly vague. You are undoubtedly interfering with permissible speech as well."[40]

There were also public condemnations against those who knew about the massacre but kept silent. Chicago mayor Richard M. Daley said it was a disgrace for people to have kept quiet about the killings. "I hope the state's attorney does a grand jury investigation on this [matter]." He emphasized that those who reportedly knew about the murders had a responsibility to come forward. "Just think about what the families had gone through, all these families who lost loved ones.... When people keep silent, I think it's a disgrace," he said. He indicated it was up to the Cook County state's attorney's office to prosecute any of the people who reportedly knew details about the murders but never told police.[41]

Referring to Luna and Degorski, Chief John Koziol hit the proverbial nail on the head when he used the phrase "typical sociopath type." Many psychiatrists consider sociopaths and psychopaths as one and the same. Sean Mactire, in his insightful book **Malicious Intent**, states:

- Before you can gain a clear understanding of how criminals think, you'll need to have a clear understanding of terms used by the criminal justice officials and by psychologists. Unfortunately these terms are often misused by the media, which can lead to errors in thinking about the makeup of the criminal mind.

There is no single way to describe criminals, especially violent criminals, nor is there any one psychiatric label that would fit their behavior. . . . With respect to violent criminals, there are two main categories that psychology, but mostly society, has deemed to fit them into. These categories are psychotic and psychopath. Again, these are labels, and unfortunately, these terms are chronically misused by the public. Frequently, these terms are used interchangeably, and too often, the word *crazy* or *insane* is used to apply to both. Both types are mentally ill.

Psychotic fits the definition of being legally insane, which is why true psychotics are a minority among violent criminals. Psychotics are out of touch with reality, and often they hear voices or see visions or both. Ed Gein, the real-life model for the main character of Hitchcock's *Psycho*, is a classic example of a psychotic. There are also a number of mass murderers who fit this category. For these demented creatures, their madness has led them to kill.

Psychopaths, or as they are often called, *sociopaths*, are quite different. Psychopaths are also mentally ill, but they are in touch with reality and therefore are not legally insane. Psychopaths know right from wrong, and they are aware that their criminal behavior is wrong, yet they consciously choose to follow a path of evil. This is not the behavior of a crazy person. Psychopaths also lack any conscience and could[n't] care less about the harm they do. To them, their crimes are many times regarded as a sport, and they rampage through society without guilt or remorse.[42]

The following morning, Saturday, both of the accused were driven from the police department to the Cook County Criminal Court Building for a bond hearing. Judge Mary Margaret Brosnahan ordered that both men be held without bond. What follows are selected excerpts from the transcript of the information given in court. Assistant state's attorney Linas Kelecious made the presentation. (Throughout this section, "Witness A" refers to Anne Lockett; "Witness B" refers to Eileen Bakalla. So as not to interrupt the continuity of the narrative, we have included some previously cited details.)

Your honor, first of all we should start out by pointing out that this is a capital case in that the defendants murdered seven people and did so during the course of an armed robbery.

They committed these murders on Jan. 8, 1993, shortly after 9 p.m. at the Brown's Chicken Restaurant at 168 W. Northwest Highway, Palatine, Ill.

The people they killed are: Michael Castro, age 16; Guadalupe Maldonado, age 47; Marcus Nellsen, age 31; Rico Solis, age 17; Lynn Ehlenfeldt, age 49; Richard Ehlenfeldt, 50; and Thomas Mennes, 32.

Defendant James Degorski: DOB: 8/20/72—age 29 now, age 20 then;

Defendant Juan Luna: DOB 2/16/74—age 28 now, age 18 then;

Here are the details of the murders:

Palatine Police Officer Ron Conley responded to 168 W. Northwest Highway on Jan. 9, 1993 at approximately 3:11 a.m. to look for an employee of Brown's Chicken who did not return home from work the prior evening. Brown's Restaurant closed at approximately 9 p.m. on Jan. 8, 1993. Upon examining the interior of that location, he discovered seven bodies in the cooler area of the restaurant. Five bodies were in the freezer that is on the east side of the restaurant and two bodies were in the cooler on the west side.

In [the] freezer were the bodies of Lynn Ehlenfeldt, Mike Castro, Rico Solis, Guadalupe Maldonado, and Marcus Nellsen. In [the] cooler were the bodies of Richard Ehlenfeldt and Thomas Mennes. Empty cash register drawers were on top of an ice machine. Subsequently, cash register tapes for Jan. 8, 1993, were totaled and compared with the money remaining in the Brown's restaurant. It was determined that between $1,800 and $1,900 in U.S. currency was missing from the restaurant.

Witness A is a 26-year-old woman and is currently a college student and is also working. She dated Degorski from 1992 ... until

1994. When she started dating Degorski she abandoned her previous group of friends. Degorski wanted it that way. He was very controlling. He was both physically and emotionally abusive to her. During her relationship with him they used to, among other things, hang out at Degorski's house. Living at the Degorski house at that time period were his mother, brother Kevin and younger sister Megan. Witness A remembers that Luna and Degorski used to torture little animals in the garage.

[She] will testify that Degorski lived in the basement in a small bedroom. He kept several knives there, along with a .38-caliber revolver. [She] knew it was a .38 because Degorski told her. She saw the gun at least three times. On one occasion, Degorski opened the gun and Witness A saw that the gun could hold six bullets. The gun, when [she] saw it, was on a crate next to the bed. Degorski would not let anyone in his bedroom without his permission. Witness A remembers one of the knives being a hunting knife with a brown handle and long blade and another knife being a switchblade.

Degorski called one day in January 1993 and told her he did something and that she should watch the news that night. The lead story ... was the murders at Brown's Chicken. Witness A called her mom and asked her to cut out the articles about the murders and bring them to her, which she did do.

Shortly thereafter, she was at Degorski's house and in his bedroom with Luna. She recalls this very vividly and has been living with this for a long time. Degorski asked her if she wanted to know what happened at Brown's. She said yes. Degorski began by telling her that he had already told Witness B, a female friend of Degorski, because they were going to use Witness B as an alibi. Both Degorski and Luna then proceeded to tell Witness A how they killed the people at Brown's Chicken. The conversation lasted a long time with each of them talking about how they did it and Witness A would sometimes ask questions.

Witness A will testify that they said that Luna really wanted to kill

someone and Degorski said that he would help. They brought
lots of bullets, "pockets full."... They continued to say how
each of them used the gun, which Degorski said was his .38, to
shoot people. It was clear that Degorski did most of the
shooting, and Degorski even talked about how Luna did not kill
one guy when he shot him, so Degorski had to kill the guy. Witness A remembered Luna reenacting how he held a woman
around her neck and at the same time cut her throat with a
knife. He said he was calling her a bitch for something she said
or did in regards to the safe, which got Luna upset.

Witness A will testify she remembered them saying they had to use
some physical force to control everyone and get them in the
coolers. [She] remembered them saying that one of the
younger guys threw up some french fries. They said they
cleaned and mopped up. Witness A also remembered them
saying something about messing with the clock. They told [her]
how much money they got but [she] cannot remember how
much. They said that they threw their clothes and shoes in separate Dumpsters. They threw the gun in the Fox River in Algonquin or Carpentersville at a place where they used to fish.
Degorski told her that he would kill her if she ever told anyone.

Other than that one time in Degorski's bedroom, Luna and
Degorski never [again] talked to Witness A about the murders.
Sometime after this conversation, [she] was at Degorski's house
when Luna called and said the Palatine Task Force wanted to
talk to him. Degorski told [her] that [she] should go with Luna
when [he'd be going] there in order to make Luna appear more
legitimate. Degorski said that they should both dress nice so
that the police would not suspect him. It appeared to Witness A
that both Degorski and Luna had talked about what Luna was
supposed to tell the police.

Witness A will testify that Luna drove [her] to the Task Force. He
was well-dressed, wearing black pants and a nice trench coat.
[She] said they sat in a waiting room until a detective came and

got Luna. No one asked Witness A any questions. Luna was back out in less than an hour. He said it was easy and that they took a photo of him.

Witness A will testify that she kept a diary for a while and documented some of these things. But she destroyed the diary for fear of getting caught by Degorski.

Witness A will testify that approximately seven to eight months ago she told her boyfriend what Degorski and Luna told her back in 1993. Her boyfriend is the first person she told. They struggled with what they should do. Her boyfriend was concerned for [her] safety. They considered sending an anonymous letter but did not. They then felt compelled to share this with another friend since he lived with them and his safety was also an issue. They obtained FOID (Firearm Owner's Identification) cards. Witness A also told her sister and another friend. Finally, [she] just recently told her mother because Degorski contacted her mother several times looking for Witness A. Witness A had to tell her mom why she had not wanted Degorski to find her. [Her] mother did give Degorski [the] phone number a couple of years ago and he called Witness A. She has not seen him since 1994 and only spoke to him that one time.

On May 9, 2002, the truthfulness of Witness A's disclosure was conclusively proven when DNA analysis conducted by the Illinois State Police Forensic Science Center revealed that James Luna's DNA profile matched the DNA profile on the chicken meal found in the garbage at the scene. This profile would be expected to occur in approximately 1 in 130 trillion black, 1 in 8.9 trillion white, or 1 in 2.8 trillion Hispanic unrelated individuals. It was further proven by the fact that she disclosed that Luna and Degorski told her that one of the victims had vomited, a detail that was never publicly disclosed.

On May 15, 2002, Task Force members interviewed Witness B and she revealed what she knew. She will testify that on the night of the Brown's Chicken homicides, she was working and got a call from Degorski. He told her to meet him at the Jewel-Osco. He said [the two men] did something big. When she got to Jewel in Carpentersville, Ill., both Degorski and Luna were there. She saw latex gloves on the [console] of Luna's car. They all got into her car. Luna [had] a canvas bag. They drove to her room-mate's townhouse in Elgin. Her roommate was out of town. En route they told her that they had robbed the Brown's Chicken in Palatine. At the Elgin residence they split the money in the bag. Witness B got $50. She thought there was over $1,000 in the bag. They smoked a couple of bowls at the Elgin residence and hung out there for about three hours. She then drove them to Luna's car at the Jewel and dropped them off.

Witness B will testify that Degorski said to drive by the Brown's. When she did they saw the ambulances and police cars. Degorski then told her what happened. Degorski told her that they went to the Brown's Chicken to rob. They first ate. Some-thing happened at the counter. They put everyone in the coolers. Degorski said that one of them started shooting, but Witness B does not remember which one. Degorski killed everyone in one cooler, and Luna killed everyone in the other cooler. Luna cut the older lady's throat. They mopped up the mess. They went out the...door. Degorski said they threw the gun in the river at Algonquin Crossing by the [dam] where they used to hang out.

Witness B will testify that the next day, she and Degorski got Luna's car and took it to a car wash. Degorski sprayed out the interior of the car. [He] focused on the front floor and the seats. A couple of days later, she and Degorski went shopping. She bought shoes with her $50. Degorski bought clothes.

On videotape, Luna said they were there to rob the place. They chose Brown's because he had worked there and knew there was no alarm. They went at 9 p.m. because it was closing time and there would be few people. He ordered a four- or five-piece children's meal and ate. They then put on latex gloves. Degorski started shooting first. They put five people in one cooler and two in the other. He recognized the owners, Richard and Lynn Ehlenfeldt, and a former employee. He shot into the cooler containing the five individuals, but claimed he did not know if he hit anyone....

It appeared that no victims had personally been robbed. The restaurant appeared to be in the final stages of closing. The floor was mopped and all of the preparation area had been cleaned. A bloody mop...was found.

In the dining room, found in a trash can (that appeared to have already been changed for the night) was a chicken dinner. The meal was partially eaten and still intact. The drink cup had never been filled. It was a do-it-yourself beverage set-up. The safe was closed and locked, with the key in the top portion. It appeared as though the top portion of the safe was empty, but on the rear shelf on the top portion more United States currency and change was left, but this was not visible without getting down low and looking inside.

The Cook County Medical Examiner's Office did the autopsies on the seven bodies; the protocol indicated that all seven deceased died from gunshot wounds. In addition, Lynn Ehlenfeldt and Michael Castro [had] knife wounds. Mrs. Ehlenfeldt's throat had been cut.

The firearms examiner for the Northern Illinois Crime Lab has received fired bullets recovered from the Brown's Restaurant and from the bodies of the seven deceased. He states that the bullets were .38 caliber and at least 11 of the bullets were fired from the same weapon; more than 20 projectiles were recovered from the scene. The positively identified rounds came from different locations. A very likely hypothesis can be drawn that all rounds came from one gun. All the bullets are soft, round-nose lead type. No shell casings were left at the scene. The rifling of the murder weapon is five right, and according to the firearms examiner, the murder weapon is likely a .38 or .357 Smith and Wesson or Ruger.

There is absolutely no doubt that they committed these murders.[43]

As for the other side, it came as no surprise that both Luna and Degorski had pleaded not guilty. Eventually it was determined that each man would be tried separately.

2002–2007

The next five years were marked by the slow-moving but intense efforts of the prosecution and the defense to shore up their cases. In 2003, state prosecutors wanted to order a foot mold of Degorski in an effort to match a shoe print found at the crime scene. Police said that the print was made by someone with a size 12 to 14 shoe, and that Degorski wore a size 12. A Cook County judge allowed the mold to be taken. In 2006, attorneys for Juan Luna brought a mass of frozen chicken to Purdue University to have it tested by a bird expert. Their contention was (1) that more chicken bones had been preserved than would have been present in the single piece Luna ate, (2) that Luna's DNA did not come from the last meal ordered on the night of the murders, and (3) that perhaps there was another chicken meal mixed in with Luna's. It was unclear to many observers how such reasoning might help the accused, yet it was another request that might have cast some doubt, and also delayed the start of Luna's trial.

Extended legal wrangling wore on—days, weeks, months filled with pretrial maneuvering over a number of issues: an attempt to suppress the defendants' statements, independent testing of Luna's DNA as well as that recovered from the chicken bones, and a reexamination of fingerprints from the crime scene.

Luna's seasoned trial attorney, Clarence Burch, sought to have the remains of the chicken meal retested to verify that the initial test results obtained in 1998 were correct. "We'd like to retest the actual chicken," he announced, "but it was a trace amount of DNA to begin with, and we don't know what's left."[44] Meanwhile, prosecutors furnished laboratory reports showing that a napkin found with the chicken meal contained fingerprints that did not match Luna's or Degorski's. "The fingerprints did not match anyone in the case," Burch said. "We're using it to negate the presence of my client. They thought this napkin was significant."[45] The attorney also stated he would challenge the methods used to collect, store, and test the remains of the chicken meal. He would even challenge my deposition regarding my involvement in the case and particularly my discovery and examination of the so-called last meal—the chicken dinner found in the garbage can. Of course, in so doing, they would have to contend with my photographs, sketches, and notes regarding the chicken bones.

And early in this period, prosecutors provided defense lawyers with computer disks containing about three hundred thousand pages of police reports, laboratory reports, and interview material that had been amassed in the ten years since the crime. Burch commented that even if he and his staff read it all at the rate of a thousand pages per week, several years would be needed to finish it all. Some predicted the trial would not start for another two years; in fact, five years would pass between the arrests and the first trial.

THE FIRST TRIAL

Juan Luna's trial began on April 13, 2007, fourteen years after the crime and five years after his arrest. During jury selection, CBS 2 legal analyst Irv Miller said of Luna's apparent videotaped confession: "[Y]ou will be able to see his demeanor; you'll be able to see the surrounding circumstances, how the police treated him, were they yelling at him, screaming at him, or did he just sit there and have a conversation and tell the police what he did?"[46]

In addition to the videotape, the prosecution was expected to link Luna to the murders through the half-eaten chicken meal and the revelations of Anne Lockett and Eileen Bakalla. But the defense was likely to argue that this was not sufficient evidence for a conviction. Referring to the defense's position, Miller predicted Luna's lawyers might exclaim:

"Attack, attack, attack ... it's not reliable, it's not him, somebody else did it." ... In the end it will be the jurors who decide his fate. The prosecution will hold nothing back and State's Attorney Dick Devine will lead the case. [They] must think they have a pretty strong [one], because the state's attorney himself is trying the case, and he's not about to put his reputation on the line if he didn't think he had a winner.[47]

Cook County Criminal Court Judge Vincent Gaughan would preside over the trial in the Cook County Circuit Court. A former public defender and supervisor for the Cook County public defender's office, he was appointed to the bench in 1991 to fill a vacancy and was elected the next year. He served in the US Army from 1964 to 1968, the last two years of which were in Vietnam. He received a Bronze Star for valor there.

Opening statements got under way on April 13, a Friday. The prosecution began by showing a videotape of the grisly crime scene. It was the first time any of the victims' relatives had seen it. Some of them, packed in the courtroom, cried in horror. Addressing the jury, Devine vowed to prove that Luna, along with Degorski, was the killer; pointed to a chicken bone in a napkin that he claimed contained Luna's DNA; showed pictures of the seven victims while indicating how they must have begged for their lives, and described each victim's wounds.

Relatives and others in the courtroom choked back tears or openly wept. Even the Palatine police officer who had discovered the bodies became flushed with emotion. He testified that upon opening the freezer door, he saw "a mass of humanity ... one body on top of each other, arms and legs on top of each other, unable to tell how many."[48]

Burch agreed that the scene was gory but emphasized that his client was innocent, that a chicken bone with Luna's DNA on it did not prove he committed the crime. "The facts are horrific," he said to the jury, "... but you promised us when we selected you that you would keep an open mind. ... It's not an open-and-shut case."[49]

On day two, Jane Homeyer testified that on January 11, 1993, two days after the bodies were discovered, she noticed all garbage cans in the restaurant were empty and clean—except one. In it she found a box that contained four chicken pieces, including a leg that had been partially eaten. Under the box she noticed three additional chicken pieces, french fries, biscuits, a cole slaw container, foam plates, and four napkins. She stated she recovered a palm print from one of the napkins (which was later matched to Luna's left palm). Under cross-examination, she acknowledged that the chicken evidence had not been refrigerated between January 9 and January 14, 1993.

Later that day, Richard Cunningham, a former DNA analyst for the Lifecode Company in Connecticut, testified that in 1993 the partially eaten piece of chicken was tested at Lifecode following my request. It did not contain enough DNA for RFLP analysis (see explanation of this procedure in the sidebar below) to link the piece to anyone. He said that consequently the bone was thrown out and explained that DNA testing technology had vastly improved since then. When cross-examined by the defense he said photographs taken of the evidence sent to him at the time were missing. (This is an obvious example of the breaking of the chain of custody of physical evidence.)

On the third trial day, Eileen Bakalla took the stand. She testified that she kept her nine-year secret out of fear. She related what Luna had told her during the morning hours immediately following the killings, a time when they both smoked marijuana. "It was almost like [Luna] was bragging about what he had done," she said. "He was smiling about it."[50] She then gave a detailed account of what transpired over most of January 9, the day after the crime.

At one point, Luna's lawyer asked whether or not she understood what Luna was saying about the crime. Burch asked, "As you sit here today you don't remember one word that came out of the lips of Juan Luna, do you?"

"No, not exactly," Bakalla responded.

Burch pressed on. "When you smoke [that] reefer, it gets you high and you see and hear things that aren't there?" he asked.

"No, it relaxes me," she answered.[51]

The fourth day of the trial—April 19, 2007—was my day to testify. The day before, I had flown to Chicago to participate in a pretrial meeting in which we discussed the case in its entirety and reviewed certain questions I might be asked when testifying. And I brought with me the original notes and photographs I had taken when examining the evidence.

As far back as 1994, when I was brought in as a forensic adviser, I was convinced that the half-eaten chicken would eventually be the key to solving the crime. I held firm to that conviction right up to the trial.

"My initial assessment in 1994 was that this was a significant finding because there was only one meal in the garbage. This individual [would] either be a witness or a suspect," I said. This was also the way I put it during my testimony in 2007. I then added, "Whoever [was] eating this meal [was] not really eating the meal.... Either something [was] wrong and they left, or [the person] was there waiting for something." I further stated that after reviewing the case, I had decided that "the most important evidence [to] pursue is the chicken," advising authorities to "try to get some DNA." And despite the somber atmosphere in that courtroom, I could not resist saying, "If a chicken place gave me a piece that small, I'd probably want my money back."[52] In addition, my original photographs of the chicken meal were used to demonstrate to the jury that the chain of custody had been made.

At that time—in 1994—RFLP was the type of DNA analysis used. A small quantity of DNA was extracted from the chicken bone, but no profile was obtained. However, things were different four years later, when the STR method was used. (See the sidebar below for an explanation of these methods.) The DNA that had been extracted in 1994 was retested and a profile was obtained. This DNA profile was entered into the CODIS DNA data bank but a "hit" was not obtained.

There have been great advances in DNA technology in recent years, and there's a world of difference in the sophistication of today's DNA analysis as compared to that of 1994. That time and 1998 are key years in the chronicling of this criminal case.

Since the DNA of every individual, with the exception of identical twins, is unique, the testing of specific portions of the DNA in biological evidence (such as saliva on the chicken bone in question) can be highly individualizing. DNA typing for identification purposes has been applied in forensic laboratories to analyze many types of biological evidence, including blood, semen, saliva, hair roots, bone, and other tissues. It has proven extremely valuable in cases such as homicide, rape, and hit-and-run accidents; the identification of skeletal remains; missing-persons investigations; and paternity issues.

DNA, or deoxyribonucleic acid, is the biological compound that contains the genetic or inheritable material of the organism. Located within the cell, DNA is present in all body fluids and structures that contain nucleated cells—that is, cells with a nucleus. Each cell contains approximately 7 billion nucleotide pairs. And what is a nucleotide pair? It is the unit from which DNA is built. Half of an individual's DNA is inherited from the mother and half is inherited from the father. The result of such recombination is that the DNA of each person is unique, except, as noted above, in the case of identical twins, who possess the same DNA. (Recent research now suggests, however, that in some instances, even the DNA of such twins may be differentiated, although the required technique currently has not been applied to forensic samples.)

Forensic DNA analysis basically utilizes the following methods:

Restriction Fragment Length Polymorphism (RFLP). This is the oldest type and requires a DNA sample of relatively good quality and large quantity. It is more difficult to work with, especially when the amount of DNA is small. This was the technique available in 1993 and 1994, when scientists were unable to establish whose saliva was on the chicken bone.

Polymerase Chain Reaction (PCR). This requires much less DNA than RFLP and is the technique referred to and used four years later (1998) in matching Luna's DNA with the DNA on the chicken bone. Using PCR, less then one-billionth of a gram of DNA can be successfully tested.

Short Tandem Repeat (STR). This most recent type of analysis has emerged as the most highly employed by forensic science laboratories. With STR, as little as 250 picograms of DNA is required. (One picogram is one trillionth of a gram.)

We would be remiss if we did not mention another type of DNA: mitochondrial DNA. In contrast to nuclear DNA, this exists outside the nucleus but is still within the cell wall. Mitochondrial DNA analysis is not as precise as, say, STR analysis, but because mitochondrial DNA does not degrade as easily as nuclear DNA, it is of particular value in cases where the sample has been exposed to the environment for long periods of time or where the sample is very old. Thus, for example, it has proven invaluable to forensic anthropologists in identifying excavated skeletal remains—even remains that are centuries old. However, because mitochondrial DNA is maternally linked it is much less informative than nuclear DNA.

After my testimony, Cecelia Doyle, a former Illinois State Police crime lab scientist, was summoned to the witness stand. She said that in 1998 she had identified DNA profiles of two people from the chicken dinner. The defense argued that the swabs used to collect such evidence were lost, as was the computer that contained the analysis. And under cross-examination by Allan Sincox, one of Luna's lawyers, Doyle said that after she had tested five swabs she was able to find at least two DNA profiles, but there could have been more. "All I can say," she stated, "is there was an indication of saliva. I got a mixture of DNA profiles. There was more than one contributor from the sample."[53] She went on to say that she could exclude two men, one of whom confessed to the crime in a 1998 video (to be discussed later). Doyle also indicated that the analysis allowed her to rule out the seven victims and eighty-one other individuals, including all investigators.

In reference to the lost swabs and computer, Sincox asked, "Every single swab taken in connection with this case have all been lost, is that correct?"

"They were sent out and never received at their destination," Doyle replied.[54] Later she said the computer and data analysis were eventually recovered.

In the second week of the trial, the thrust of the prosecution's case was what most expected; there were no bombshells. Key elements were:

- For the first time, scientists linked Luna to the crime scene with fingerprints and DNA evidence. DNA expert Kenneth Pfoser employed statistics to implicate Luna through DNA analysis. "It's a match," he said categorically. "The DNA profile would exclude [all but] 1 in 139 trillion blacks, 1 in 8.9 trillion Caucasians, and 1 in 2.8 trillion Hispanics."[55] Mark Lyon, one of Luna's lawyers, attempted to shoot holes in the testimony by referring to the human genetic code, asserting that Pfoser's analysis covered only a fraction of the code.
- Then fingerprint expert John Onstwedder linked Luna's left palm print to a partial print on the napkin found in the trash bin along with the chicken meal. Luna's print was taken upon his arrest in 2002 and compared with a photograph of the print found on the napkin. The scientist used a slide presentation to demonstrate how fingerprints and palm prints are formed in a fetus and can later be matched to an adult. "My conclusion," he said, "was that

the latent imprint from the photograph was made by the person who made the palm print."[56]

- Dr. Edmund Donoghue, a forensic pathologist, testified that all seven victims died of gunshot wounds to the head and that one, sixteen-year-old Michael Castro, was shot six times. In addition, he was stabbed in the abdomen after he died.

- Retired firearms expert Robert Wilson said he found bullets in cardboard boxes and jars of gravy, and under soda machines at the crime scene. He informed the jury that approximately twenty bullets were recovered from the victims' bodies and the restaurant itself.

- Eleven days into the trial, the prosecution's key witness, Anne Lockett, took the stand. She spoke of her relationship with Luna around the time of the slayings. She said she was seventeen then, abused drugs and alcohol, and suffered from bouts of depression. She stated Luna and his friend James Degorski had given her a detailed account of the crime and their role in it, but fear kept her silent for nine years. In 2002, however, she contacted the police about her secret. "The guilt I had ... outweighed my fear," she said evenly, "and I felt I owed it to the families. I had tried to block it out to forget about it."[57]

- Lockett testified that on that January 1993 night in question, she was in a mental hospital after trying to kill herself by overdosing on cold medications. Degorski, she said, phoned her there and suggested that she watch television because the murders would be the lead story. Then, after her discharge, the two men admitted to her that they were the killers and, in step-by-step fashion, described the crime with all its gory details. She stressed that Degorski warned her to keep silent. "If I ever told anyone anything, he would kill me," she said.[58]

- On cross-examination, Luna's lawyers tried to discredit Lockett's recollection of events, citing her history of severe depression and drug abuse. And they peppered her with the same question: If she were so afraid of Degorski, why did she keep dating him for months after the crime?

- The next day, Wednesday, the prosecution played the dramatic forty-four-minute videotape depicting Luna calmly admitting that he and Degorski committed the murders and then describing the gruesome details involved. Among other things in the video, he told police about the chicken meal that preceded the crime, about forcing the seven victims to lie on the floor before being herded into the cooler and freezer, about his slitting Lynn Ehlenfeldt's throat, and about Degorski's doing most of the shooting while he guarded the doors. In rebuttal, the defense contended that Luna's confession occurred after nineteen hours of questioning and during a time when he was kept away from his family.
- The prosecution rested its case the next morning after calling relatives of the victims to the stand as well as scientists who stated they could match Luna's left handprint and his DNA to evidence found at the crime scene (on the napkin and the chicken meal).

When the defense had its turn that Thursday, there were again no bombshells:

- Although several police officers took the stand to outline their findings on the night of the killings, much of the defense's initial hours of testimony dealt with witnesses attesting to Juan Luna's fine character, among them his brother and the manager of the restaurant in question. The brother, Jorge Luna, was the defense's first witness.
- From the very beginning the defense team tried to divert attention away from Juan Luna as the murderer by insisting that someone else was responsible. They pointed to a fingerprint that did not match Luna's on a green service tray on top of a garbage container—the same container in which prosecutors maintained investigators found the chicken meal and a napkin containing his DNA and left palm print.
- The defense referred to the partial footprint behind the counter that did not match Luna's, any employee's, or any investigator's. It

also underscored what the defense claimed was mounting evidence of a botched crime scene investigation.

- The defense alleged that Luna was abused during his nineteen-hour interrogation and that he made up the confession because (a) he wanted to see his five-year-old son (who was taken from him at the time of his arrest and brought home) and (b) he was led to believe that the police planned to pin the crime on Degorski.

- A Palatine police officer on the stand described the footprint behind the counter, another bloody footprint that didn't match any known subjects, an apparent bullet dent in a metal fryer hood, and a definite bullet hole in one of the plastic strips covering the walk-in cooler. The defense held that the dent and the hole were described in detail by another man who had confessed to the crime but who had been released by the police.

- A Chicago Field Museum scientist, a bird expert, testified that he did not wear gloves or work at a sterilized table when he examined the chicken dinner. He also said he had not written a report about his findings. His testimony was one in a series of examples the defense used to portray the investigation as slipshod. It was around this time that some members of the media began intensifying their criticism of the prosecution's case. They pointed to mislaying, mishandling, and inadequate testing of evidence; forgetting to take certain handprints; and losing copies of important interviews. "These are examples of incompetence," said Leonard Cavise, a professor at DePaul University College of Law. "It's not the kind of thing you expect from a 21st-century police department."[59]

- The defense hammered away, attempting to discredit the prosecution's case. For instance, it called on anatomic pathologist Dr. Malcolm Goodwin to support its contention that the slit across Lynn Ehlenfeldt's neck was made *after* a fatal gunshot wound to her head, not *before*, as Luna had said.

- A police sergeant testified that he took a detailed and accurate confession of the crime from a man named John Simonek in 1999. The defense showed a thirteen-minute video in which Simonek implicated himself and a friend in the killings, but the prosecution countered by labeling the confession blatantly coerced.

- DNA experts were at odds to the very end of testimony, when rebuttal witnesses were allowed to be recalled. For the prosecution, Ranajit Chakraborty, who helped develop the national DNA database used by law enforcement, said that any person off the street would have a 99.999 percent chance of being excluded as a match to the DNA in the chicken sample. This contradicted earlier testimony from a defense expert who stated that the DNA profile on the meal could appear in 1 million other people in the United States. And, in a return to the neck wound controversy, Dr. Mitra Kalelkar from the Cook County Medical Examiner's Office said that Lynn Ehlenfeldt's wound was inflicted before her death, not after, as a defense expert had testified earlier.

Testimony ended on Thursday, May 3, 2007, the trial judge announcing that closing arguments would be heard on Wednesday, May 9.

In those closing arguments, prosecutors highlighted the following facts:

- Luna plotted the robbery because he wanted to do something big.
- Luna and his friend James Degorski planned to murder everyone inside the restaurant so that there would be no witnesses.
- They decided to commit the robbery at closing time because there would be plenty of cash and little resistance.
- Luna's videotaped statements were very incriminating. Prosecutors asked jury members to "look at his gestures, look at his face ... there's no doubt he was there. His body language convicts him beyond a doubt."[60] Observers stated the prosecution attorneys stressed Luna's body language because they wanted the jury to disregard another videotaped statement from the earlier sus-

pect, John Simonek. They claimed he gave a false confession after being coached by Palatine police.

- DNA material on the partially eaten chicken meal matched Luna's DNA and linked him to the crime.

On the other hand, the defense attacked the prosecution's case, zeroing in on what they claimed was faulty handling and interpretation of DNA evidence. They also sought to plant seeds of reasonable doubt about the credibility of several prosecution witnesses. And regarding the question of videotaped body language, lead defense attorney Burch argued that if Simonek's confession was false, then so was Luna's; if Simonek was coached, then so was Luna.

"Luna uses words like east, west, and north to describe what happened," Burch said to the jury. "You think Luna talked like that? No way; he was led."[61]

Both sides did agree on one point: that facts, not emotions, should influence the jury's deliberations. As Cook County assistant state's attorney Scott Cassidy put it: "If you feel sympathy toward these victims, we want you to put it out of your mind." Defense attorneys issued a similar sentiment: "Don't get caught up in the emotional part of it."[62]

CBS 2 legal analyst Irv Miller said, "Clearly, the prosecution has the overwhelming amount of evidence in this particular case.... Degorski's forthcoming trial will involve different evidence. There isn't that [forty-four-minute] videotaped confession, and that's the big difference between these two trials. [But] it's not going to help him."[63]

The jury received the case at 3:30 p.m. on that same Wednesday, was dismissed a little more than two hours later, and resumed deliberations the next morning. All told, they deliberated only eight hours before rendering a verdict: guilty on all seven counts. He was determined eligible for the death penalty.

The same jurors reconvened four days later for that phase of the case and, because of a lone dissenter on the jury panel, Luna was spared the death penalty. About three months later, he was sentenced to life in prison without parole.

On August 31, 2009, jurors were expected to hear opening statements in Degorski's trial.

MURDER IN THE SACRISTY

I f fourteen years seems an unusually long time between a crime and its adjudication—as we have just seen in the Brown's Chicken case—consider a time span nearly twice as long. The following, which occurred in Toledo, Ohio, involved a nun, the victim of a brutal murder with ritualistic overtones; allegations that the Catholic Church was involved in a cover-up; and the eventual arrest of a priest twenty-four years after the crime—the same priest who had conducted the nun's funeral Mass.

The tragic players in this bizarre story are the nun, the priest, the Catholic Church, and Satan. Each stands out, perhaps Satan more than the others. Devil worship and evil ritualistic practices are part and parcel of the case. But let's first examine the facts.

THE CRIME

Based on recorded interviews; official forensic, medical, and police documents; and published news accounts, the following represents the most likely sequence of events on April 5, 1980. It was a cloudy Holy Saturday morning—the day before Easter—and the day before the victim's seventy-second birthday. She was Sister Margaret Ann Pahl, the sacristan of chapels at Mercy Hospital in downtown Toledo. As such, she was the official in charge of the sacristy, the room where all sacred vessels, vestments, and other church objects were kept.

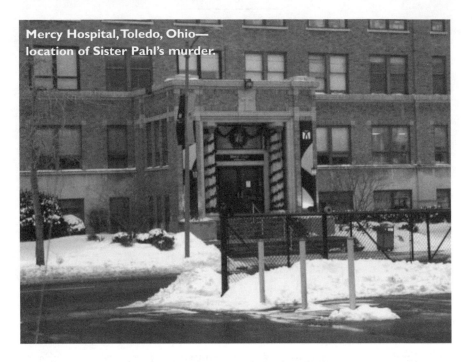
Mercy Hospital, Toledo, Ohio—location of Sister Pahl's murder.

As we shall see, many individuals crossed paths with both the victim and her suspected murderer, Father Gerald Robinson, on that early morning. This is a rare time in the Catholic calendar when no 6:00 a.m. Mass is held. But there would be an Easter Vigil Mass that evening, and, as was her custom each year, Sister Margaret Ann would be removing religious artifacts from the chapel altars. It was considered a sign of mourning for the crucifixion of Jesus Christ.

Significantly, she was still smarting from a disagreement she had had with Father Robinson on Good Friday—the day before. More than one person later attested to her having confided in them about it and to her uncharacteristic display of emotion over the issue. It was not the first time the nun and the priest had clashed over matters both administrative and religious. By all accounts, he—thirty years her junior—considered her to be domineering in their discussions. The chaplain also purportedly resented having to repeat various instructions to her because her hearing was failing, as was her memory for details.

Author John Glatt wrote in his excellent book *Forgive Me, Father*:

At noon on Good Friday, April 4, 1980, Father Robinson said Mass
in [the] chapel, with Sister Margaret Ann Pahl among the small
congregation. A few hours earlier, the Holy Eucharist—the
body and blood of Jesus Christ—had been placed in [the] sacristy. In *the* most solemn service of the year, Catholic tradition
dictates a series of meditations and readings, as well as the
highly dramatic Passion account from the Gospel of St. John,
involving the priest and the congregation.

But today Father Robinson inexplicably shortened the service,
without consulting anyone else. Sister Margaret Ann Pahl
became so indignant, she challenged him on it.

As the elderly nun berated him, Father Gerald Robinson remained
silent, merely staring at her through thick black-rimmed
glasses, before walking out of the chapel, leaving her distraught
by [the] altar.

"I think this was the final straw," Lucas County Lead Prosecutor
Dean Mandros later claimed. "A lot of things had been building
with him over time. And he just snapped."[1]

Within minutes, Sister Margaret Ann spoke with housekeeper
Shirley Lucas, who usually judged her as "on the cold side." Lucas was
stunned when the nun squeezed her hands and, with tears in her eyes,
said, "Why do they cheat God out of what belongs to him?"

"I lost it," Lucas recalled. "I cried after she turned around. I had to
go to the bathroom. I don't know if it was because it was the first time
that she ever touched me and held my hand. She just looked so pitiful
and emotional. Maybe she had a feeling that something was going to
happen to her."[2]

On Holy Saturday, Sister Margaret Ann's day began at 5:30 a.m. She
showered and then donned the traditional Sisters of Mercy habit: blue
smock with a cross pinned on the left side over a white long-sleeved
blouse. She left her seventh-floor dormitory room half an hour later,
taking the elevator down to the first floor, and greeted Sue Bentley at the
switchboard. Moments later she was in the sisters' dining area in the cafe-

teria and conversed briefly with Audrey Garraway, an employee there. Sister Margaret Ann exited the cafeteria carrying a green food tray, went directly to a supply closet in the hallway, and placed a stack of cleaning cloths and a container of incense on the tray. She evidently had emptied the tray in the chapel before Garraway saw her reenter the cafeteria with the same tray and order a breakfast of grapefruit, raisin bran, and coffee. Audrey recalled that the sister appeared preoccupied with her thoughts as she picked at her meager meal, then left in a hurry and headed for the chapel. On the way the nun passed two ambulance drivers, employees of the hospital, who were coming off the night shift. One of them, Jerry Tressler, remembered checking his watch. It was 6:50 a.m.

Sister Margaret Ann's exact movements over the course of the next ten minutes are unclear (she was, after all, alone at the time). In any event, the best guess is that she entered the sacristy at approximately 7:00 a.m. Whether or not her assailant was hiding in wait or entered seconds later is also unclear.

Forty-five minutes later, Sister Madelyn Marie Gordon, the chapel's organist, knelt down in a pew to say her morning prayers before preparing to arrange the music for the evening's service and to help Sister Margaret Ann clean the altar for the accompanying Mass. Already there, Sister Mary Phillip was praying, to be joined later by Sister Clarisena. When Sister Madelyn Marie was finished, she walked to the organ, shuffled through some music sheets, and realized that she was uncertain about one selection for the service. She thought she had better consult with Father Robinson about the matter and would call him on the phone in the sacristy. It was situated just to the side of the chapel. She checked her watch. It was 8:20 a.m.

Sister Madelyn Marie was puzzled when she found the double doors to the sacristy locked; she had glanced in that direction when she entered the chapel only minutes earlier and they were open. She used her own key to open them and walked into the dimly lit room.

She saw what she initially assumed to be a CPR dummy lying on the tile floor, but on closer inspection it turned out to be Sister Margaret Ann. Sister Madelyn Marie stiffened in horror and stood momentarily speechless as she stared at the body's swollen face and the sliver of blood on its forehead. The younger nun's eyes drifted over the scene rapidly, and she noticed that the elderly nun's habit was up near her breasts and her girdle and panties were down at her ankles. In the next split second, she observed Sister Margaret Ann's arms were positioned close to her sides and her legs were straight and close together. She would later testify that her immediate impression of the body's position was that it had been posed on the floor as if part of some strange ritual, and she believed that the blood on the forehead represented a weird anointment.

The organist raced out screaming that Sister Margaret Ann had been raped and murdered. She then sobbed uncontrollably in Sisters Mary Phillip's and Clarisena's arms.

A more official description of the victim at the scene of the crime is contained in an early report of lead detective Arthur Marx:

> The body was positioned as follows: head to the west, feet to the east. Her veil, which is black in color and worn as part of the Sister's uniform, was lying under the back of her head, with the end of the veil extending out and to the right.
> There were visible traces of what appeared to be dried blood on the bridge and tip of the nose. There were also numerous puncture type wounds on the right side of the face. The blood that apparently seeped from these wounds appeared to still be wet and was dark in color.[3]

Marx also alluded to a white altar cloth from the chapel that was wrapped around the victim's right forearm and extended down along the right side of her body to just below her knee. He further stated that because her hands were positioned with their palms up, she had probably not been able to defend herself, and he noted that her eyeglasses lay on the floor about eight inches from her right hand. He also observed that she was wearing a "blue jumper-type knit dress" that had apparent stains on its front. He went on to write:

> The stains were concentrated above the left side of the upper chest. The dress was saturated with the stains, which were still moist. Numerous punctures were also visible in the dress in the area of the upper left chest.
>
> The victim was also wearing a white long-sleeved blouse, gray panty hose, a white rubber elastic panty girdle that had been pulled down and was now resting around the right ankle. The girdle would have been slid over the left ankle and foot to be found in this position. The victim was also wearing blue Oxford type shoes (laces both tied).[4]

With respect to Father Robinson's possible behavior just before and around the time that the crime took place, investigators and prosecutors would later theorize—both among themselves and at the trial—that he had been seething with anger over his most recent confrontation with Sister Margaret Ann. What's more, that he was tired of her controlling attitude. They assumed that the previous night, all night long, he tossed and turned, his mind in overdrive.

And in fact, yes, he was her murderer. Familiar with the sister's routine, he devised a plan. It had elements not only of killing her, but also of a satanic version of performing her last rites and—by virtue of the pattern of the stab wounds he positioned over her heart—inflicting the ultimate degradation on a person whom, he felt, deserved no less. But there would be more. He would insert a crucifix into the virginal nun, an act representing yet another "ultimate"—the ultimate defilement of Sister Margaret Ann's vows of chastity.

Prosecutors would speculate that he rose at about 6:00 a.m., and after showering and putting on his black cassock and a pair of rubber-soled shoes, he removed a letter opener from a desk drawer and placed it in a duffle bag. Dagger-shaped, the opener had been presented to him by his Boy Scout troop after returning from a trip to Washington, DC.

Arriving at the chapel door at approximately 7:00 a.m., he stole in and tiptoed to the entrance of the sacristy. Once assured that Sister Margaret Ann was working there, he returned to the chapel door and locked it. He spotted a long white linen cloth near the altar and, picking it up, moved cautiously into the sacristy. His prey was standing on a chair removing drapes, her back to him. When she stepped down from the chair, he went at her, slinging the cloth around her neck from behind, pulling and twisting it. She was immobilized quickly, but he kept on with the choking. Who knows what feeling he was experiencing? In the process, he had fractured the hyoid bone in her neck and caused tiny blood vessels in her eyes and face (called petechiae) to rupture.

He laid her lifeless body on the floor and began his warped last anointing, this time to the devil himself. He covered her with the altar cloth and placed a crucifix—upside down—over her heart, using it as a template for what was to follow. Removing the letter opener from his duffle bag, he thrust it into her body around the edges of the crucifix. There was only a small amount of blood, for by that time her heart had stopped beating. Next, he stabbed her repeatedly about the face, neck, and chest—thirty-one times in all. When he saw that some blood had surfaced on the handle of the opener, he pressed it forcefully on her forehead—enough to leave an imprint.

Then, in an additional act of blasphemy and humiliation, he pulled her habit up over her brassiere, lowered her undergarments, spread her legs, and, unspeakably, penetrated her—albeit slightly—with the very same crucifix he had used as the template.

His carefully planned attack completed, he must have smiled devilishly as he stood to view what he had done. In a final calculated gesture, he straightened her legs and arms and neatly posed her bloodied and half-naked body, hoping the whole undertaking would be taken as a ritualistic message to the glory of Satan.

Now, to repeat—this was the scenario that prosecutors would eventually put forth. The reasoning behind each facet of the ghastly incident, even the identity of the perpetrator himself, might have been open to question, but the brutal findings were real—and there for all to see.

BACKGROUND OVERVIEWS

Father Gerald Robinson

Gerald Robinson was born on April 14, 1938, in Toledo. His mother, Mary Sieja, had emigrated to America from Poland, and John, his father, was of German descent. John was a laid-back man who was a custodian in the local school system, in charge of furnace maintenance. It was Mary's insistence that set the family's traditions as Polish. She also helped point her son in the direction of the priesthood. On the way, Gerald eagerly absorbed the details of Polish culture and learned to speak its language.

He enrolled in St. Mary's Preparatory High School in nearby Orchard Lake, Michigan, a highly respected training ground for Polish American boys who wished to become Catholic priests. It wasn't long before he could recite—without missing a beat and with obvious reverence—the school's mission to anyone who would listen: "To provide deserving young men the moral guidance, discipline, and education necessary to become Christian gentlemen, scholars, and men of service and leadership for the world." In retrospect, one wonders how long he would remember those words.

Robinson next studied at S. S. Cyril and Methodius Seminary for four years and was ordained a priest in 1964. Five years later, St. Mary's was honored to have Karol Cardinal Wojtyla visit the campus. He would later become Pope John Paul II.

From the moment he was ordained, the quiet, reserved Father Robinson was idolized by Toledo's close-knit Polish community, a feeling that never seemed to diminish, even during the scandal that arose forty years later. Many of them believed he had been cast in the mold of all priests, none of whom could do any wrong.

From a more objective perspective, most of his career seemed spotty, even shadowy. He was often deemed moody, introverted, and unpredictable. There were sudden transfers from one parish to another and more than a few unexplained demotions. Of a more serious nature were the following:

- He was accused of the ritual abuse of two girls, one at Toledo's St. Adalbert's Church during the period between 1968 and 1975, and the other at Toledo's Mercy Hospital in 1978. The alleged victim in the latter episode would come forward in 2003 to help resurrect the Sister Margaret Ann Pahl case. Though her accusation was unsubstantiated by diocesan officials and investigators, her complaint no doubt precipitated an intense police investigation that led to his arrest and indictment.
- A vague report suggested he was a member of a group connected to another ritual abuse of a female. Its members, who called themselves the "Sisters of Assumed Mary" (SAM), were Toledo men who did what they termed "nun drag" (wearing nuns' clothing) in Toledo churches.
- Before the 1980 murder, his demotion to third-rank priest at St. Michael's Church appeared to indicate that the diocese was aware of some problem.

Sister Margaret Ann Pahl

Margaret Ann Pahl was born on April 6, 1909, in the rural hamlet of Edgerton, Ohio. Her Roman Catholic parents were of German heritage and were devout churchgoers. Francis, her father, was both a farmer and a carpenter. Margaret Ann grew up without running water, electricity, or indoor plumbing—but with plenty of love from her parents and eight siblings. Some believed it was her spartan upbringing that prepared her well for the simple religious life that was to follow. In school she was studious, outgoing, and ambitious, and there was probably never a doubt that she would become a nun. She was perhaps inspired by two cousins who were in the Sisters of Mercy order. Early on, she would often proudly announce her intention to follow in their footsteps.

After high school, she spent a year at a retreat center first as a postulant, then a novice, absorbing all she could about religious life and the Mercy order. Thereafter, she earned a bachelor of arts degree from Toledo's DeSales College, and from 1930 to 1933 she made her initial and then final vows. In between she began nurse's training and received an RN degree from St. Rita's Hospital in Lima, Ohio.

Distinguished supervising and executive positions followed at numerous Ohio Mercy Hospitals. Sister Margaret Ann took her increasing responsibilities in stride and was once described as a devoted jack-of-all-trades who tackled everything in the hospital building except engineering.

In 1971, at age sixty-one, Sister Margaret Ann considered retirement—but only briefly. Instead she asked for and was given the responsibilities of sacristan at Mercy Hospital, where her attention to detail was legendary—and where she eventually suffered a violent, inhumane death.

"She demanded everything to be done exactly as she wanted it, and on time," one homicide detective wrote after interviewing a nun who called her "old school." One hospital worker told the same detective, "She was distraught because...the chapel was not as perfect as she wanted it."[5]

Toledo Diocese Cover-Up?

So why did it take twenty-six years to prosecute Father Robinson? He was, after all, the prime suspect from the start. Some law enforcement officials pointed to a lack of sufficient evidence that could be used against him. Others claimed a priest was not capable of such a heinous crime. However, there was also a lingering suspicion that a diocesan cover-up was responsible, and that it applied to other cases, including instances of priest involvement in pedophilia and other deviant sexual activity. Some analysts considered the Robinson episode to be the poster child for protection of the priests of the Catholic Church, at least in the Toledo area. But there was another aspect to this case that the church evidently wanted to squelch: The murder had satanic rite written all over it. Many contended that some church officials would rather have had the public believe that sexual assault alone was at the heart of the crime.

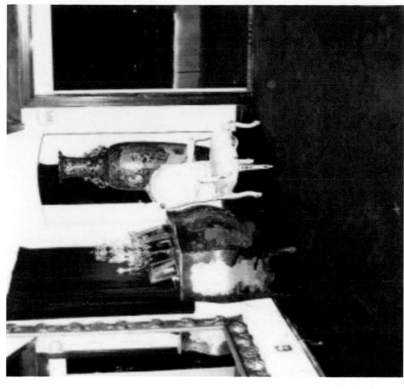

Same scene after police released it thirty-eight hours later.

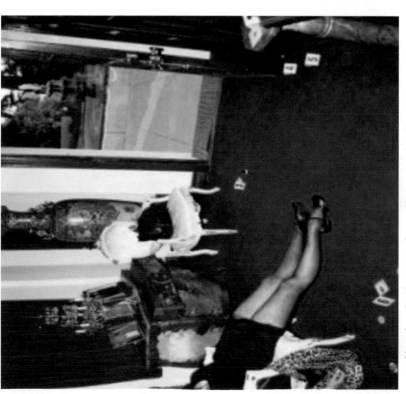

Shooting death scene after police arrived at Spector's home.

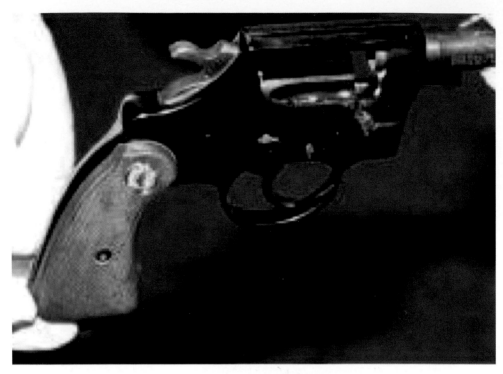

Spector's gun showing blood and tissue.

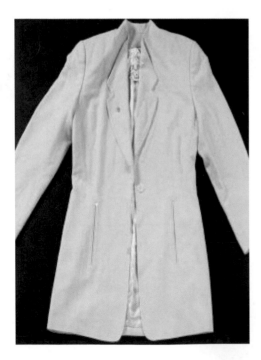

Spector's overcoat with only a few bloodstains.

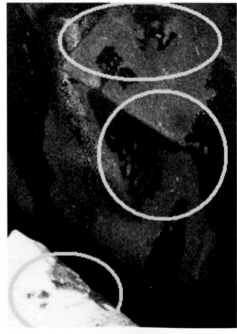

Clarkson's dress with a large amount of blood spatter.

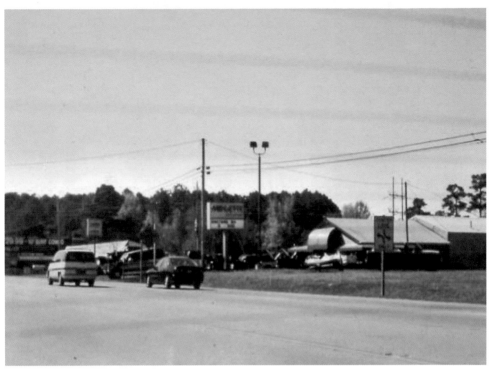

Location of Brown's Chicken & Pasta restaurant.

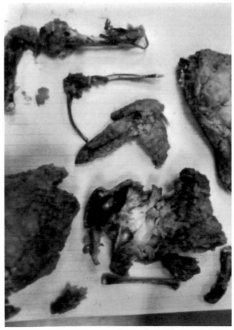

```
------------- 21:07----
4FCHTY/D        5.29
   INDFRY       0.00
   INDSLW     : 0.00
SM DRINK        0.89
*DINE IN       -0.00
TAX1            0.51
TOTAL         6.69
CASH          10.00
0001A         21:08
```

Cash register receipt in Brown's Chicken massacre case.

Chicken meal in Brown's Chicken massacre case.

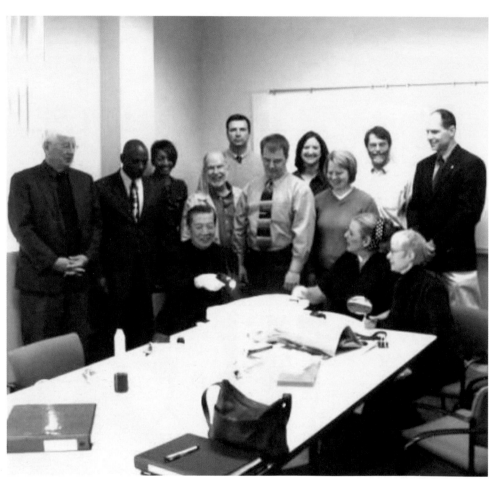

Task force meeting with Dr. Lee in the Sister Pahl case.

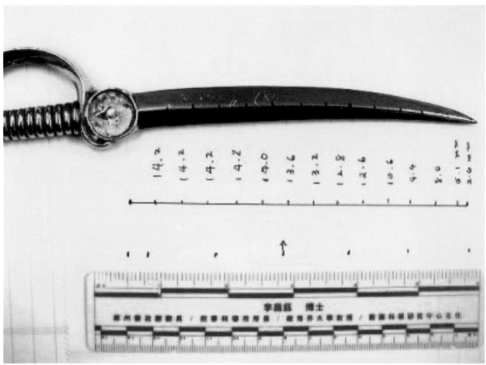

Letter opener used as murder weapon in the Sister Pahl case.

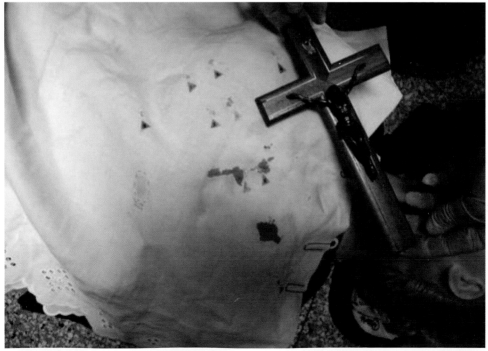

Stab wounds through the altar cloth, forming a distinct upside-down shape of a cross in the Sister Pahl case.

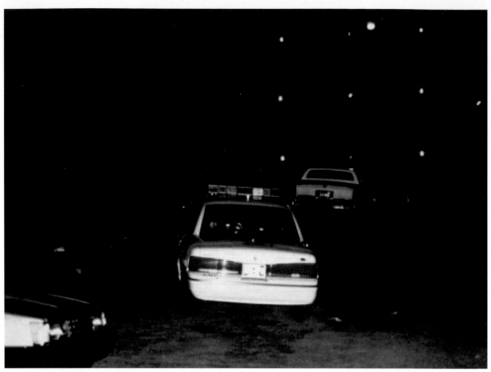

Officer Allan's cruiser behind the white Cadillac in a vacant Hartford lot.

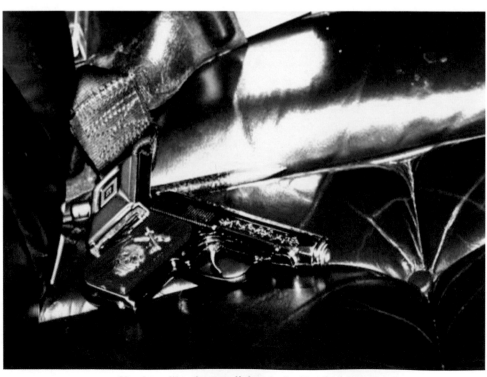

Handgun-like cigarette lighter in the Hartford case.

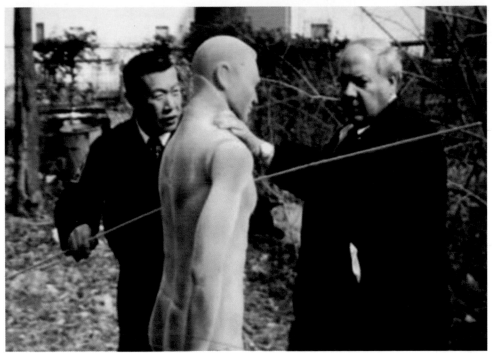

Dr. Lee and State Police Lab assistant director Kenneth Zercie reconstructing the bullet trajectory in the Hartford case.

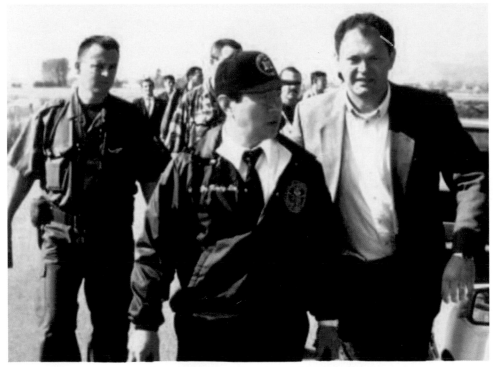

Dr. Lee and Dr. Andelinovic arriving in Bosnia.

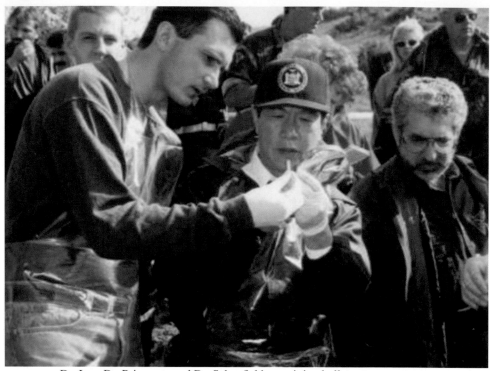
Dr. Lee, Dr. Primorac, and Dr. Schanfield examining bullets at a mass grave.

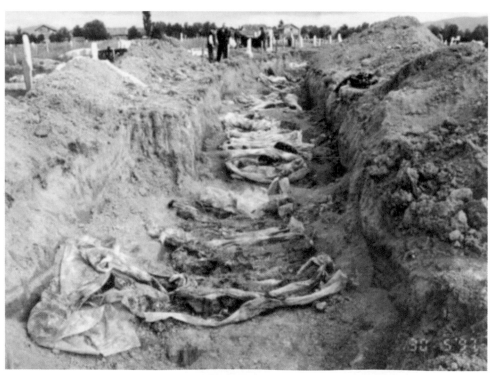
One of the mass grave sites in Bosnia.

The following few snippets no doubt constitute the tip of the iceberg in lending credence to claims of impropriety and injustice. They raise doubts about the sincerity of certain elements within the church and about fairness within the Toledo criminal justice system.

- The deputy chief in charge of the investigation, Ray Vetter—a devout Catholic who publicly asserted that priests and nuns were "next to God"—had detectives continue typing police reports in triplicate (the normal procedure), but instead of distributing them in the usual manner, ordered that they all be sent to *his* office.[6]
- Dr. Renate Fazekas, the physician who performed the autopsy, said the body was left in a staged position and that there had been no indication of rape or any other type of sexual assault. ("Sexual assault" as it is defined today would include the insertion of an object into the private parts. In this case, the object would refer to the crucifix, not the letter opener, which was the murder weapon.) Lieutenant Bill Kina, the detective who interviewed Fazekas about her findings, added, "This was done, as far as I'm concerned, only to defile [the victim]."
- But the lieutenant saw a general lapse in the criminal justice system when it came to sexual matters. "There was an unwritten rule. When you caught a priest in a homosexual or a pedophile situation, you didn't book them like you did any other individual. You took them down to the vice squad, who then called in the Monsignor. He'd then come down and put a collar on them and take them away and do whatever was appropriate with the church at that time."[7]
- As part of the investigation, which we shall examine in more detail later, Kina and Detective Art Marx were in the so-called Safety Building interrogating Father Robinson when Vetter, Monsignor Jerome Schmidt of the Diocese of Toledo, and Mercy Hospital attorney Henry Herschel interceded. After spending ten minutes alone with the priest (in the absence of

Kina and Marx), they herded Robinson out of the building. Shocked, Kina turned to speak with Father Jerome Swiatecki, the other chaplain at Mercy, who had witnessed the entire incident. Kina asked, "Where are they taking [Father Robinson]? What are they going to do with him?" Swiatecki responded, "They'll put him on a funny farm somewhere and you'll never hear from him again."

- "There was a lot of steam taken out of the investigation when they pulled him out of there," Kina recalled twenty-six years later. "We later found out Deputy Chief Vetter had gone down to the diocese to pick up Monsignor Schmidt and bring him down to the Safety Building. He brought the attorney along to take care of the police. . . . I don't think he was trying to protect or justify the killing of a nun. He was trying to protect the sanctity of the Church. Even today I don't think you could get him to admit he did anything wrong, because he was such a devout Catholic. . . . He thought he was doing right."[8]

- A little more than a year later, Kina, still exasperated at the shielding of his prime suspect so close to a confession, decided to retire from the police department after twenty-nine years of service. "I felt that the job was getting me down . . . and morale was very low. I mean, you don't give anybody, including priests, a carte blanche ticket to do anything they want. Now running a red light, I can see looking the other way, so you don't get a priest involved. But as far as homicide, you don't give anybody a green light to just go ahead and carry on with their life after that."[9]

- It wasn't only the "looking the other way" that rankled many in law enforcement, it was the method used. Many still contend it was the first time in American history that a monsignor of the Catholic Church had interrupted a police interrogation.[10]

- But Kina's resignation was not the only one possibly influenced by the aftermath of the murder. John Anthony Donovan, the bishop of the Catholic Diocese of Toledo, had been considered meticulous in handling all diocesan affairs. Four months after the murder, he suddenly resigned. More than a few observers wondered if he suffered from pangs of conscience, but whatever the reason, no other bishop in the diocese had ever resigned from his post.[11]

- Because of increasing nationwide reports of sexual abuse by priests, a national victims' advocacy group called Survivors Network of those Abused by Priests (SNAP) was founded in the late 1980s. Claudia Vercellotti, herself a victim of clerical sexual abuse, was SNAP's organizer in Toledo. Once the organization was in place there, a special church review board was appointed to hear abuse allegations. Its membership consisted of five Catholic laypersons and one non-Catholic.

- Twenty-nine-year-old Sister Annie Louise (not her real name), who taught children with special educational needs in Catholic schools in and around Toledo, began to suspect that she had been sexually abused as a child by clergymen in strange robes. She was certain she had repressed any memories of the incidents and decided to seek counseling.

- It should be noted that not all "repressed memories" turn out to be accurate or true. They can even be inadvertently implanted in the mind by a well-meaning therapist. However, in this case, specifics about the encounters emerged gradually, particularly the name of her main abuser, Father Chet Warren. Unknown to her, five other women had already accused the priest—who had been expelled from the Oblates of St. Francis de Sales—of similar abuse. But she remembered a second abuser: Father Gerald Robinson! It took more than ten years for the nun's experiences to crystallize, and at that point she contacted Vercellotti. Details of the nun's experiences will be described later, but for now, in the context of assembling examples of a possible church cover-up, suffice it to say that Sister Annie Louise was invited to appear before the review board.

- The day before her appearance, she presented each board member with a four-page single-spaced typed statement about her ordeals and mentioned Father Robinson by name. The statement began: "This report is written for the Diocesan Review Board members to chronicle the severe abuse I experienced, beginning at age two."

- The meeting itself was long and emotional for the nun, who recounted all she could remember about the years-long abuse. She then left the room at the Catholic Center while the panel deliberated. Dr. Robert Cooley, a psychologist specializing in sexual abuse and the one non-Catholic on the board, demanded that her allegations be brought to the police immediately, but the rest of the board disagreed and his demand was voted down.

- "We suspect that this was an effort to 'contain' the information ... on Robinson," said Vercellotti. "The Toledo Catholic Diocese should have laced up their gym shoes and sprinted over to the prosecutor's office. But they didn't."[12]

- In the mid-2000s, a fire of suspicious origin broke out in Vercellotti's apartment, destroying eighteen file drawers of research and insider documents. Most of the documents pertained to cases of priests allegedly abusing minors.[13]

- At about the same time, a retired Toledo police detective spoke candidly about the special relationship between the department and the Catholic diocese. "I can tell you there was always somebody the diocese could go to in the police department," he admitted to the *Toledo Blade*. "And I can tell you that, at one time, I was that man."[14]

- Listings in the *Official Catholic Directory* are most revealing, carrying with them certain implications. After the murder in 1980, Robinson was made pastor at Polish parishes *without* schools and a decade later, the *Directory* listed him in residence at two parishes *with* schools and administrator at a third parish. The implication could be made that, during that period, his assignments were better accepted by classifying him as "in residence" or "administrator" at a particular parish. It would be some time before he would assume a hospital position like his ill-fated one at Mercy Hospital.

Satanism, the Black Mass, and Ritualistic Sexual Abuse

"Satanism," "the Black Mass," and "ritualistic sexual abuse" are terms that bear indirectly on this case. They refer to subjects poorly understood by some and shunned by others. First, some definitions:

- Satanism is the worship and imitation of the biblical Satan or Lucifer. It is the antithesis of Judaism and Christianity. There are two kinds of Satanists: (1) those who believe that Satan exists and is a powerful force, sometimes sacrificing animals and children as a means of worshiping him and obtaining his favor, utilizing the Black Mass as the main rite; and (2) those who believe he does not exist but is merely the symbol of fleshly human desires and appetites, which they try to emulate through a variety of sins, pleasures, and perverse activities.
- The Black Mass is the ultimate rite for a real Satanist to gain magical (though of course imagined) powers. It is a blasphemous Mass in which the altar is a nude woman and the vagina is the tabernacle. Usually, a real Host—or in some cases a crucifix—is stolen from the Catholic Church and is inserted into the vagina while participants recite distorted psalms interspersed with obscenities, curses against Jesus, and honors heaped on Satan. The rite usually ends with the fake priest having real sex with the "altar." Thus the Black Mass combines various elements, including the belief in a pagan deity stigmatized by Christians as the devil, the use of the Mass for personal ends—especially sexual in nature—and the parody of orthodox Christian ritual. It is obviously an inversion of the Catholic Mass and often involves human torture and sacrifice.
- Ritualistic sexual abuse can range from saying prayers in a sexually abusive context to the manipulation of a sacramental environment (such as sexual solicitation during Confession) to full-blown satanic ceremonies, including the Black Mass. Victims of this type of abuse are often reluctant to make allegations because

of the whispered denial that nuns and priests could contemplate such activity, much less participate in it. Why those initially committed to a godly life could turn their sworn faith completely on its head and succumb to evil, we'll leave for others to ponder.

The allegations of two Toledo women will illustrate the relevance of these types of acts in the Sister Margaret Ann Pahl murder case. The first involves the aforementioned Sister Annie Louise, who wrote and spoke of her ordeals before the review board and whose cause was defended by Claudia Vercellotti; and the other, Jean Marlow (also not her real name).

Sister Annie Louise outlined how Father Chet Warren molested her at her home while her mother rested upstairs. She gave graphic descriptions of continued sexual abuse over the next few years and her eventual recruitment, along with other members of her family, into a satanic cult. She stressed that its rituals were "horrifying and sadistic," and that they were "designed to break our wills and internalize whatever core programmed message they wished to use to further our powerlessness."

She wrote that at about age five, she was taken to a cemetery and placed in a coffin. "Cockroaches were released into the box," she stated. "[T]hey told me the bugs were marking me for Satan."

She related explicit details of members of the cult (called The Circle of Darkness) initiating her to the slow beat of a drum as she was carried to a table by a priest and vaginally raped; of being penetrated by a snake "to consecrate these orifices to Satan"; of witnessing the killing of a three-year-old child and being left alone with the little girl's mutilated body for hours in "a sea of blood and stench"; and of being forced to eat an eyeball at the age of eleven. "They wanted me to know they were always watching me."

She indicated that when she was fourteen, Father Warren had pimped her out to men for sadomasochistic sexual liaisons. "One of these S&M perpetrators was Father Gerald Robinson, a diocesan priest," who, she said, paid to have at least one encounter at St. Vincent Hospital.[15]

The kind of behavior described by Sister Annie Louise is an almost textbook definition of ritual abuse. In his fine book *When Satan Wore a Cross*, Fred Rosen put it this way:

> Ritual abuse involves the sexual, physical, and psychological assault on a victim, by one or more "bad guys." The idea is to bring a ritual to fruition, thus satisfying the demands of the deity in question. It's important to understand that... ritual abusers see nothing wrong with what they are doing. They are doing it to fill some inner, warped need. Since children are society's most defenseless individuals, ritual abusers target kids who can't fight back.[16]
>
> Jean Marlow's story was not unlike that of Sister Annie Louise. In 2005 she accused Father Robinson, who was one of her early childhood teachers, and his friend, a lay preacher, of being members of a cult of priests who wore nuns' habits and performed satanic rituals. As noted earlier, they were known as the "Sisters of Assumed Mary." In civil court papers, Marlow, now in her early forties, alleged that she had been the victim of "clerical ritual and sexual abuse" from her preteens onward, naming Robinson and other clergy, who, she wrote, would dress up in "nun drag" and subject her to vile atrocities in the name of Satan. Upon seeing photographs of her alleged abusers in the newspaper, she began to piece together her horrible nightmare and decided to go public with claims of rape, oral sex, sodomy, torture, and forced participation in animal sacrifices.
>
> "They cut [me] with a knife as a sacrifice to Satan," Marlow's civil suit stated, "and drew an upside-down cross on [my] stomach. They forced me to drink the blood of a sacrificed animal."[17]

The Investigation

There are two investigative phases to consider in this case: early and late. Actually, very late—a quarter of a century late. The early stage

obviously involved the period immediately after the crime, a time when
Father Robinson became everyone's main suspect. This was fueled by an
early comment made by the other chaplain at Mercy, Father Swiatecki.
As he was performing the last rites on the victim in the sacristy, Father
Robinson walked in. His face was expressionless, his eyes blank. The
hospital's emergency code had been broadcast over the public address
system a short time before, calling all medical personnel to the sacristy.
Several house staff doctors, student nurses, nuns, and others responded.
Father Robinson was an exception; he had to be summoned down from
his second-floor quarters by the hospital administrator. Everyone
assembled in the sacristy knew of the exception, and as they observed
the last rites ceremony, they also saw Father Swiatecki rise from his
knees and angrily confront Father Robinson. "Why did you kill her?" he
asked, his voice trembling. "Why did you kill her?"[18]

The Toledo Police Department was informed of the murder at
about 8:30 a.m., and within minutes, several detectives and an evidence
technician arrived at Mercy Hospital to investigate. There followed the
usual cordoning-off and processing of the crime scene, along with
interviews of possible witnesses. There was not one.

The Autopsy

Late that day, Lucas County assistant coroner Dr. Renate Fazekas performed the autopsy. The narrative, in part, is as follows:

> The body is that of a 71-year-old female weighing 134 pounds and
> measuring 62 [inches] in length. The body is dressed in a blue
> sleeveless dress...white blouse, blue under slip, white bra,
> pantyhose, girdle pants, and blue shoes. Pantyhose and girdle
> pants are gathered around the ankles. A black veil accompanies
> the body.
> A silver-colored necklace, with a [silver] cross attached is around
> the neck. A [silver] cross is pinned to the left side of the dress.
> A silver cross ring is on the 4th finger. Rigidity has not yet

developed. Lividity [is] absent. [Lividity is the postmortem discoloration of the skin due to settling of blood in dependent parts of the body.]

A 3½ [inch] long oblique [appendectomy] scar is over the right lower abdomen.

A 1½ [inch] long oblique scar is over the medial aspect of the left knee.

The teeth are natural.

The body is involved with multiple stab wounds and evidence of strangulation. There are six stab wounds to the left side of the face. The stab wounds are transverse and oblique over the left angle of the mouth and just below the left side of the jaw. The deepest penetration measures 1½ [inches].

There are fifteen transverse and slightly oblique stab wounds to the left aspect of the neck. The direction of the stab wounds is from front to back. The deepest penetration measures 3 [inches].

There are nine transverse and oblique stab wounds to the left side of the chest, between the left clavicle [collarbone] and nipple line. Two of the stab wounds range in size from 1/8 [inch] to ½ [inch] in length. They are similar to the above described stab wounds. Some have a slightly irregular outline. The direction of the stab wounds is from front to back. The deepest penetration measures 3 [inches].

The left common carotid artery [large artery on the left side of the neck that carries blood to the head] reveals a rent at the cranial segment [within the skull]. The larynx and trachea reveal three stab wounds. The esophagus is perforated one time. The fourth and fifth cervical vertebrae are each involved with a stab wound. The entire anterior and lateral neck is hemorrhagic.

Her left lung had been stabbed twice.... [T]he sternum contains stab wound at the level of the third [intercostal] space, which extends through the right ventricle [of the heart], just below the cusps of the pulmonary valve.

[Evidence of strangulation]: Numerous distinct petechiae [minute round hemorrhages] involve the conjunctiva [mucous membrane covering the exposed surface of the eyeball and which also lines the inner surface of the eyelids] of both upper and lower eyelids and the face with the exception of the forehead. Both supra and infraclavicular areas [areas above and below the collarbone] are recently bruised (blue). The area measures 10 [inches] by 4 [inches]. An oblique linear bruise, outlining the necklace, is over the right supra and infraclavicular area.

Both cornu of the hyoid bone [the horn-shaped ends of a small bone in the neck] are fractured. The fracture sites are surrounded by hemorrhage.

A 3½ x 2 [inch] recent bruise prominently involves the bony ... area of the lower cervical and upper thoracic spine, slightly to the right. Within the area are three parallel longitudinal, linear bruises, each measuring 2 [inches] in length.

[Cause of Death]: *This 71-year-old white female, Sister Margaret Ann Pahl, died of multiple—31—stab wounds to the left side of the face, neck and chest. There was also evidence of strangulation.*

Also mentioned in the autopsy report is the doctor's opinion that the murder weapon had a blade at least three inches long and half an inch wide. It had four sides, with a cross-section resembling the shape of a kite or a diamond.

Fazekas also called attention to the fact that there were no defensive wounds, that there was a small scratch inside the vagina, and that the hymen was intact with no evidence of penetration. (Evidently the crucifix was not inserted in that far. Rape kit results also indicated that no semen was present in vaginal, oral, or anal orifices.)

What was *not* reported however, either by the doctor or earlier by the detectives, was that the nine stab wounds over the victim's heart formed the pattern of an inverted cross.[19]

Key Items/Issues

Four days passed after the murder and no substantial evidence—such as fingerprints, footprints, fibers, or hair—turned up. Moreover, no weapon was discovered. Then, in what Kina believed to be a turning point in the case, housekeeper Shirley Lucas described Sister Margaret Ann's deeply emotional reaction to Father Robinson's intention to shorten Good Friday, Holy Saturday, and Easter Sunday services. This is where the nun's comment of exasperation came in, as noted above: "Why do they cheat God out of what belongs to him?" Recall that Sister Margaret Ann had confronted the chaplain about his decision to pare down the services. Was this all tied in with a motive? Robbery had been ruled out, for nothing was missing from the sacristy or chapel. And there were no signs of male penetration.

Several developments during this early phase merit comment: a keen assessment by Kina, the recollection by a witness of footsteps described as fast and frantic, the discovery of a likely murder weapon, a "sighting" by a medical resident, a fake confession, and a polygraph test. None of these alone incriminated the chaplain, but taken together they made a strong case for his complicity. At best, they could be grouped as circumstantial. However, that was not enough, since suspicious activity—even widespread—does not add up to guilt.

We will now address these developments one at a time.

First, a consultation with the assistant coroner helped to convince Kina that Sister Margaret Ann had not been murdered by a stranger.

"The victim knew her assailant," he explained. "A stranger would not have killed the victim in such a vicious manner. It would take somebody with a very strong vendetta to go in and kill a person in that ferocious manner. I mean, if a stranger comes in and his intention is to rob or rape the victim, he's going to stab them once or twice, or maybe cut their throat. But he's not going to stand there and stab them thirty-one times."[20]

Then, a week after the murder, Mercy Hospital receptionist Margaret Warren told Detective Dave Weinbrecht she had heard loud, rapid footsteps overhead in the professional building on Holy Saturday morning. She stated it was about 7:30 a.m., and that just before, she had encountered janitor Wardell Langston as she made her way to her reception desk. Langston told her that he had heard strange steps when he was cleaning carpets under a balcony by the main entrance.

"[It sounded like] something was terribly wrong," he later told the detective.

Both Warren and Langston indicated that the footsteps came from the area of Father Robinson's quarters. Both also said they had not heard the clang of the heavy panic bar (a horizontal bar on a door that may be pushed to open the door in an emergency) at the end of the overhead hallway, but that the step noises appeared to stop in the vicinity of the chaplain's door.

"[Warren] described the footsteps as being very rapid and frantic," Weinbrecht wrote in his report. "They started westbound from the hallway that comes down from the bridge and turned left...to the point at the end of the L-shaped hallway in front of Father Robinson's quarters. These footsteps excited and scared [her]. She thought they were frantic."

Informed of the footsteps and the fact that both observers' stories jibed, Kina was impressed. "That was significant," he said. "They fell within the timeframe of the homicide. The balcony and the entrance to the nurses' quarters is actually where the priest lived. And he [Langston] heard frantically running footsteps up on the balcony and running down that hallway to Robinson's room."[21]

Two weeks after the murder, Father Robinson signed a waiver of search warrant, allowing detectives to search his two rooms at Mercy Hospital. It was then that they found a dagger-type letter opener in a desk drawer. Measuring eight inches long, it had a diamond-shaped blade, a knuckle guard at the lower end of the handle. It bore a circular bronze medallion on the handle with an embossed picture of the US Capitol building. In all of its details, it fit Fazekas's description of the murder weapon.

A few days later, the letter opener was examined by Josh Franks, senior criminalist at the Toledo crime lab. "It was sumptuously clean,"

Franks noted. "It didn't have any fingerprints, no stains, no smear marks. It appeared as if it had been polished, and that was interesting."[22]

Franks pried off the medallion and found a small spot on the underlying surface. He tested the spot for blood using phenolphthalein, a chemical used for the presumptive test for blood. The result was positive. But there was not enough of the substance remaining for a confirmatory test, and the presumptive test alone would have limited evidential value in court.

Detective Dan Foster interviewed Dr. Jack Baron, a thirty-two-year-old second-year medical resident who was one of the first to respond to the emergency call over the public address system. He said that as he rushed down the stairs, he took a wrong turn because he had never visited the chapel before. He turned back and passed a priest in a black cassock. Baron said the priest glanced back, giving him an icy stare. He described the priest as being between thirty-five and forty-five years old, of medium height with brown hair—all of which described Father Robinson.

Then, during one of two interrogations, Robinson suddenly claimed that Sister Margaret Ann's murderer had confessed to him, a revelation that shocked both Kina and Marx. They knew that if it were true, the priest had violated one of the Catholic Church's cardinal rules: that a priest must never disclose anything about a confession and that such a violation is punishable by automatic excommunication.

"He says, 'I'll tell you what happened,'" remembered Kina. "One of his parishioners had come in and confessed to killing the nun, and he took his confession." When pressed on the issue, especially with respect to the confessor's identity, Robinson threw up his hands and admitted he had made up the story because he wanted to protect himself. He also said he was exhausted and simply wanted to go home.

"Here's a Catholic priest [who] would lie to the police during an interview," Marx explained years later. "He said, 'Oh, I just made that up.' That's critical."[23]

Finally, about two weeks after the murder, Father Robinson was given a lie-detector test in the detectives' bureau interrogation room.

He later admitted he had taken Valium earlier that morning. Lieutenant Jim Weigand administered the test.

In his official report, Weigand indicated that Robinson had contradicted himself several times during the questioning and that he was possibly lying through portions of the procedure. Weigand concluded in his report: "Truthfulness could not be verified.... Deception was indicated on relevant questions concerning the murder of Sister Margaret Ann Pahl."[24]

The Hiatus

For the next week or two, virtually nothing of any consequence emerged. This meant that the investigation had stalled in less than a month. Detectives gave their own perceptions of the situation with comments such as "We're at the bottom of things to do" or "The handwriting's on the wall" or "For all intents and purposes, the investigation's at a standstill" or "It's damned stressful, that's all."

The accumulated circumstantial evidence—supported by the continued efforts of a trimmed detective staff in addition to an increased monetary reward fund—all seemed to go nowhere. The investigation droned on for several more months, even a year or two, and then fizzled into a cold case. Nonetheless, at Mercy Hospital rumors persisted that the homicide was part of a satanic rite and that Father Robinson was the killer. And the detectives once active on the case all agreed, one saying that the clergyman possessed the elements of the key triad—motive, opportunity, and means—"in spades."

Nearly twenty-five years would pass before the case would heat up again. In the interim Father Robinson resumed his duties at Mercy, but approximately fifteen months after the murder he was reassigned as pastor of three Polish churches: St. Anthony, St. Stanislaus, and Nativity. Eight years later, he was appointed associate pastor of St. Joseph Church in Sylvania, but within six months was transferred to a part-time ministry at Flower Hospital and Lake Park Nursing Home. At that time he resided at St. Hedwig Parish.

"He lived at my rectory for four years," said Father Paul Kwiatkowski, the then parish priest at St. Hedwig. "He's a very shy and quiet person—like a Caspar Milquetoast in a way. A bit of a pushover and wishy-washy."[25]

Later, in semiretirement, Robinson performed pastoral care at nursing homes and hospitals around Toledo. And on weekends he preached at various churches around Toledo.

One Sunday in the early 1990s, Detective Art Marx walked into church and spotted his one-time murder suspect conducting Mass. "And I'm not walking up to the Communion rail," he remembered. "I'm leaving church early."[26]

CASE REOPENED

In late 1997 newly appointed Lucas County Prosecutor Julia Bates, impressed by the use of modern DNA technology in the exoneration of Sam Sheppard for the murder of his wife in Cleveland, decided to utilize the new technology in the evaluation of old cases under her purview. She and her associates achieved success in finally bringing closure to several cold cases. Two years later, her department joined forces with the Toledo Police Department to form a permanent cold case squad whose mission was to reinvestigate old cases by using DNA and other new technologies. Its members included Detective Tom Ross, a very seasoned investigator with the prosecutor's office; Sergeant Steve Forrester, one of the best detectives in the Toledo Police Department; Assistant Coroner Diane Scala-Barnett; world-renowned forensic anthropology experts Drs. Frank and Julie Saul; and members of the DNA Team from the Bureau of Criminal Investigation and Identification (BCI) in Bowling Green. They began holding monthly meetings and, over a period of seven years, examined fifty cases and resolved about thirty. But Sister Margaret Ann's murder was not among them—not yet, anyway.

Then, as a consequence of Sister Annie Louise's coming forward with her accusations, as well as the dogged efforts of Claudia Vercellotti from SNAP and the influence of Forrester and Ross from the cold case squad, the 1980 murder case was officially reopened in December 2003. It had, in effect, lain dormant for almost a quarter of a century.

The first order of business was to look at the evidence that had been stored in the police department's property room. Two particular things stood out: the dagger-shaped letter opener and the altar cloth. The two detectives unfolded the large altar cloth and noted a long, thin, dried bloodstain. They then compared the shape of the opener's blade and handle with the bloodstain and believed it to be almost a perfect match, a significant blood transfer pattern. They took it a step further by consulting with Dan Davison, a forensic scientist at the Ohio Bureau of Investigation, and the best he could conclude in his report was that he could not include or exclude the opener as the potential murder weapon. It was a minor disappointment, but it was at least a start to the reinvestigation—they had gotten the ball rolling.

They next interviewed Sister Annie Louise. In the course of their discussion, the nun asked if the victim had been stabbed in the shape of an upside-down cross. They found the question significant, for the detectives were well aware that this was a detail Sister Annie could never have known if she were not credible.

The biggest obstacle in reopening the case was that some of the Toledo Police Department's reports had disappeared, including those dealing with Father Robinson's interrogations and an interview with Father Swiatecki, who had died ten years before. But Detectives Bill Kina and Art Marx were still alive—hovering around eighty—and the two diligent cold case detectives were in direct contact with Ross and Forrester. Gradually, faded memories became more focused, and soon the prosecutor's office hosted regular roundtable discussions involving the four detectives and a prosecutor's representative.

"Some of those early meetings [with Kina and Marx] were just introductions," said Forrester. "Just to tell them what we're doing and what we're about. See what they remember."

"All these reports were missing," said Kina. "So we didn't have anything to go on as far as the priest's involvement in this, other than our memories... [and the roundtable sessions were] the only way it was resurrected. It brought all this stuff back."[27]

Acting Bishop Michael Billian couldn't help much either. In response to a request for Father Robinson's diocesan personal records, the bishop turned over a file. Later, Forrester wrote:

> The file was substantially devoid of any information concerning Father Robinson's service in ministry... [his] performance evaluations (or their equivalent), and/or any internal (canonical) investigation(s) conducted by the Catholic Diocese of Toledo into the death of Sister Margaret Ann Pahl or Father Robinson's fitness to serve in ministry.
>
> In short, the Catholic Diocese of Toledo provided information concerning Father Robinson, which included [only] his picture, brief biographical information, his date of ordination and bare-bones information concerning his service in ministry.[28]

In January 2004, the cold case squad arranged to have DNA testing performed on Sister Margaret Ann's underclothing. A small amount of DNA was found, but DNA experts reminded investigators that *anyone* in contact with the body during the initial investigation could have contaminated it.

Still, the renewed investigation seemed to be gathering steam.

Deputy Coroner Diane Scala-Barnett concluded that the letter opener could have caused the stab wounds.

Detective Terry Cousino, assigned to the Forensics and Crime Scene Unit of the Toledo Police Department, demonstrated that a certain bloodstain on the altar cloth—a transfer pattern—was consistent with the curve and shape of the tip of the opener's blade. In addition, he pointed out other consistencies involving parts of the letter opener, along with bloodstains and puncture holes in the altar cloth. He would later testify about these findings.

T. Paulette Sutton, a famous expert in bloodstain pattern analysis, and Father Jeffrey Grob, the archdiocese's exorcist and occult expert, were consulted, and both provided valuable information—as we shall see later.

Finally, with the flurry of endless interviews and scientific analyses concluded, DA investigator Ross arrested Father Robinson on an aggravated murder charge on April 23, 2004. The arrest, made twenty-four years—almost to the day—after the crime, took place at the priest's home. As Ross led Father Robinson away, Forrester lingered behind to conduct a brief search of the home. In the bedroom he discovered a large cardboard box containing hundreds of photographs of corpses in coffins, some dating back many years, others relatively recent. And in a bookcase he spotted a pamphlet titled *The Occult*, which was published before the murder. Forrester skimmed through it and found several paragraphs underlined, including one that made the detective swallow hard. It dealt with a Black Mass in which "an innocent" becomes an altar while torture, sexual abuse, and even murder are used for satanic empowerment.

Five hours later, Father Robinson was formally charged and taken to the Lucas County Jail. The arrest warrant was succinct:

> The defendant, Gerald J. Robinson, caused the death of the victim, Sister Margaret Ann Pahl, with the cause of death being strangulation. Sister Margaret Ann Pahl was found to have numerous post-mortem cuts on her body and an instrument, with unique characteristics associated with Sister Margaret Ann Pahl's post-mortem cuts, was found to be in Gerald Robinson's possession.[29]

Reaction to the arrest was swift. Most of the Toledo Polish community was outraged. National newspapers carried the story under blaring headlines, and it made all three major television networks' morning shows. Within a day or two, it was featured in papers around the world, including England's *Daily Telegraph* and France's *Le Monde*. Prosecutors hastened to explain that there was enough evidence to charge Robinson with the murder, stating that after investigators analyzed blood patterns, they concluded that the murder weapon was the letter opener, which had been in his "control" at the time of the murder.

Less than a week later, the *Toledo Blade* printed a hard-hitting editorial critical of the Diocese of Toledo for its handling of the case, especially in view of the church's more recently publicized problem with pedophile priests:

> The diocese invited more public bruising, more disdain from communicants, and worsening assessments of its credibility by keeping bad behaviors secret until [they] become public in a shocking manner. The arrest of Father Robinson by Toledo police makes that point.
>
> Forthrightness and good citizenship are necessary if the diocese doesn't want to keep conveying the impressions of subterfuge, cover-up, and irresponsibility that have plagued Roman Catholicism here and in Western Europe for nearly two decades of sex scandals.[30]

Within a month, Robinson was released after his many supporters raised sufficient funds to post bail. Meanwhile, several former police officers began to speak openly about the case, alleging that Robinson was never arrested back in 1980 because the local diocese thwarted the investigation by putting pressure on investigators to stall their work.

On May 3, 2004, Lucas County Prosecutor Julia Bates signed the formal indictment of Father Robinson. Afterward she explained, "I saw him as a man who killed a woman...and so he happened to be a man wearing a collar, and she was a woman wearing a habit. It was a crime. We didn't look too much beyond that to say, 'Gee whiz, we better not do this, because after all, he's a priest.'"[31]

In the period between the indictment and the trial, developments that would eventually play a role in the upcoming trial were (1) the exhumation of Sister Margaret Ann's body for purposes of reautopsy and (2) my agreement to join the prosecution team and conduct a crime scene reconstruction.

I was first contacted by Dr. Frank Saul. He and his wife, Julie, have worked as a team on many cases and participated in many South American anthropological explorations together. I have known them for about thirty years through mutual lecture engagements, working on forensic cases, and exchanging ideas at meetings of the American Academy of Forensic Sciences. They solicited my assistance in this case, and Bates subsequently called and wrote to me. After considering all aspects of her presentation, I decided to take a look at this very cold case.

In the summer of 2004 I was giving an advanced homicide investigation course in Wisconsin. Cousino and an assistant prosecutor traveled there to meet with me. They brought along the altar cloth and the letter opener. During a lunch break we examined both items. I noted that the blood pattern on the altar cloth had faded over the years; however, there were still many interesting blood patterns that warranted enhancement. That December I flew to Toledo to meet with task force members and experts assigned to the case and to conduct further examinations, including a careful examination of all crime scene and autopsy photos. Then, accompanied by Forrester and Cousino, I went to the chapel to reconstruct the scene of the crime. I should point out that a CPR dummy was utilized for reconstruction and that although some of the furniture pieces were different, the floor tiles were still the same as in 1980. We were, in fact, able to reposition each piece of evidence in its original position based on the floor designs.

The next day I conferred with several forensic experts and investigators in the medical examiner's facility and, utilizing the heme-enhancement chemical tetramethylbenzidine, we sprayed the patterns on the altar cloth to enhance the bloodstain patterns.

On July 17, 2005, I issued an official report of my reconstruction of the case as follows. The referenced photographs are not all included in this book, but mention of them is retained since they were an integral part of the forensic investigation. Furthermore, reproduction of the report in its entirety serves to illustrate the meticulous nature of the process. To avoid duplication and provide balance, some details that appear in the report have been thus far omitted in our discussion of the case, since they will be covered later in this chapter, in the section concerning the trial.

RECONSTRUCTION REPORT
SUBMITTING AGENCY: Julia R. Bates
Lucas County Prosecuting Attorney
Lucas County Courthouse, Suite 250
Toledo, Ohio 43624–1680
VICTIM: Sister Margaret Ann Pahl
CASE #: State of Ohio v. Gerald Robinson
CR 04–1915
Toledo Police Department, RS#020565–80
PLACE OF INCIDENT: 2221 Madison Avenue
Toledo, Ohio
DATE OF INCIDENT: 04/05/80
DATE OF REQUEST: August 27, 2004
DATE OF REPORT: JULY 17, 2005

At the request of Julia Bates, Lucas County Prosecuting Attorney, Dr. Henry Lee of the Forensic Research and Training Center agreed to assist in the investigation into the 1980 homicide of Sister Margaret Ann Pahl. This assistance would include a review of submitted documents and materials, a crime scene reconstruction, and examination of specified pieces of physical evidence.

On August 27, 2004, Dr. Lee met with personnel from the Lucas County Prosecuting Attorney's Office and Toledo Police investigators regarding this case. On 12–28–04, Dr. Lee traveled to Toledo and conducted an examination of the scene located within the chapel at Mercy Hospital. On 12–29–04, Dr. Lee had the opportunity to examine a few items of evidence including the altar cloth and [dagger letter opener] seized in conjunction with this investigation. These items were examined at the Lucas County Examiner's Office in the presence of the Toledo Police Department's Evidence Unit.

ITEMS SUBMITTED:

Reports from Lucas County Coroner's Office, Autopsy report dated April 5, 1980

Reports from Regional Forensic Center, Memphis, TN

Reports from Toledo Police Department

Assorted B&W crime scene photographs

Re-autopsy report and copies of color exhumation process, dated 05/20/2004

Report of Forensic Anthropologists Drs. Frank and Julie Saul, dated 06/08/2004

Reports of Regional Forensic Center, by Paulette Sutton, dated 07/16/04

Report regarding Examination of Evidence, dated March 23, 2004

INTRODUCTION:

On April 5, 1980, Sister Margaret Ann Pahl was found dead in the Chapel of Mercy Hospital in Toledo, Ohio. She was lying on the floor in a supine position with apparent stab wounds to the neck and upper torso, and had an altar cloth draped around her right arm. An autopsy conducted by Dr. Renate Fazekas concluded that Sister Pahl died of multiple (31) stab wounds to the left side of the face, neck, and chest. There was also evidence of strangulation.

On May 20, 2004, the remains of Sister Pahl were exhumed and subjected to a second autopsy. Dr. Scala-Barnett stated that in her opinion the weapon in question, a dagger letter opener with the Washington, D.C., insignia, or an instrument identical to the size and shape of the weapon, caused the stabbing wounds in Sister Pahl. Dr. Frank Saul and Dr. Julie Saul also examined the exhumed remains of Sister Pahl. They concurred, and concluded that this letter opener (or another strong instrument with identical characteristics at the tip) is consistent with having produced the punctures in the mandible [lower jawbone], manubrium [upper part of breastbone], and seventh cervical vertebrae of Sister Pahl.

REVIEW OF PHOTOGRAPHS:

Photograph #1 is an overall view of the chapel within Mercy Hospital where the body of Sister Pahl was located on April 5, 1980. Photograph #2 is an overall view of the same general area as depicted in Photograph #1 as it was on 12/28/04. Note the consistency in the area as depicted 24 years prior.

Photograph #3 is a view of the doorway leading to the small room where Sister Pahl was found. This room is located off the main chapel with the door wide open. A portion of the body was seen with her feet pointing to her right. Photograph #4 depicts this area on 12/29/04.

Photograph #5 is an interior view of this relatively small room. Photograph #6 is a view of this room as of 12/28/04. Although furniture has been changed, the basic room and floor remain the same.

Photograph #8 is an overall view of Sister Pahl's body. She is in a supine position on the floor. White cloth fabrics can be seen adjacent to her right side, across her right lower leg, and adjacent to her left leg. Blood-like stains were noticed on the altar cloth and on her upper chest area.

Photograph #9 is a frontal view of Sister Pahl's body. A pair of eyeglasses is lying on the floor to the right of her right hand. There is a large bloodstain on the upper front portion of her dress. A white altar cloth is around her right arm. Blood-like stains are visible on this altar cloth, particularly the portion of the cloth furthest from her head. Blood-like stains may also be observed on her right hand.

Photographs #10 & 11 are close-up views of Sister Pahl's head and upper torso. A blood-like stain is observed on her forehead. A blood-like drip pattern is running downward on her nose. In addition to the large amount of heavy bloodstain pattern on the upper portion of her dress, blood-like spatters are observed on her dress as well as on the altar cloth located around her right arm. A hat-like object was noticed under her head. Blood smears were observed on her left cheek area.

Photograph #12 depicts a view of the white altar cloth that was spread over her right arm. A set of small defects or holes was observed on this cloth. These defects are symmetrically formed, as well as in pairs.

Photograph #13 and 14 are autopsy photos. Photograph #13 shows the frontal view of her upper body. Numerous stabbing wounds were observed on her face, neck, and upper chest areas. Photograph #14 is a closer view of the stab wounds. Note the unique cross-over configuration of some of these wounds. These wounds were more likely inflicted by a small pointed sharp instrument.

Photographs #15 & 16 are closer views of the floor which had been in the room where Sister Pahl was found. It was learned that these floor tiles were never replaced and were in their original condition. The floor tile had a textured design surface. A macroscopic examination of the tile surface was conducted and the results compared with the original crime scene photographs. Based on the tile texture designs we were able to verify that those tiles were in fact original tiles and in their original location.

A few original scene photographs depicting the floor area around her head were examined further. It was found that there were a few spots on the floor that are not part of the tile texture design. These spots are consistent with blood-like spatters. These blood-like spatters are consistent with having originated during the stabbing of Sister Pahl with her head located in that position on the floor.

EXAMINATION OF PHYSICAL EVIDENCE

Outer garment/dress. Blue in color:

Photograph #17 is a view of the upper portion of her garment. The defect holes have been marked with white reinforcement rings. A total of 21 holes was found. There is some blood-like spatter located adjacent to the bottom right portion of the heavy bloodstain on the upper chest area of this dress. A few blood-like stains are located on the inner, top, back portion of this dress. The blood patterns suggest that either the dress was pushed up before Sister Pahl was stabbed, or the victim was in an upright position as the blood was deposited downward. Examination of this dress with an Alternate Light Source revealed two areas in which there were stains exhibiting fluorescence. The nature of these stains is not known at this time.

White slip-like undergarment:

Photograph #18 is a view of the upper, front portion of this garment. The defect holes have been marked with white reinforcement rings. A total of 26 holes was found. There were more defects in the white undergarment than in the outer blue dress. One examination of this fact is that the white undergarment had been folded or bunched together, so that a single stabbing event could have produced more than one hole.

White altar cloth:

Photographs #19 & 20 depict this white altar cloth with blood-like stains and defect holes. There were 18 marked holes observed and marked with blue circles, as shown in photograph #21. These 18 marked holes were in two groups of 9 holes on each side as mirror images of each other. This fact indicates that the altar cloth was originally folded together during the stabbing. A total of 9 stabs was inflicted which produced 18 symmetric holes. When comparing the relative sizes and locations of these holes to those holes observed in the blue dress, it was found that some of the holes are in relative alignment while others clearly are not. Thus, it is likely that this altar cloth was in close contact with the victim's upper chest for a portion of the stabbing. The other wounds were likely inflicted without the altar cloth present. Further, since there is a relatively small amount of bloodstain present on this cloth in the vicinity of the holes, it is likely that the stabbings which penetrated the altar cloth, dress, and her chest occurred before the substantial flow of blood from the victim's wounds began. Several bloody contact transfer patterns were observed on the altar cloth. Some of these stains are consistent with having originated by direct contact with a bloody object in a static manner. Other patterns are consistent with dynamic movement after contact with a bloody object.

Photograph #22 is a close-up view of the handle portion of the letter opener, adjacent to a contact transfer on the altar cloth. Photographs #23 & 24 are close-up views of the blade end of the letter opener adjacent to another contact transfer located on this cloth. A bloody print enhancement reagent, Tetramethyl-benzidine (TMB), was used to enhance patterns on the altar cloth. Photographs #25 & 26 depict those patterns after enhanced by TMB.

The letter opener consists of a variable width blade, ribbed handle, with a circular medallion piece at the junction of the blade and handle. Figure #27 is an overall view of this letter opener.

CONCLUSIONS:

The small room adjacent to the chapel…where the victim was found, is consistent with a primary crime scene. Witnesses last saw Sister Pahl in the chapel, preparing for Easter Sunday Mass. She was most likely attacked in this small room, and assaulted on the floor.

Based on the original autopsy report, the cause of death was multiple stab wounds in conjunction with strangulation. External examination revealed 31 stab wounds located about the left side

of the face, left side of the neck, and left side of the upper
chest. In addition, there was evidence of strangulation as indicated by petechial [tiny, usually round] hemorrhages of the
eyelids and face, contusions [bruises] in the neck region, and a
fractured hyoid bone [*U*-shaped small bone in the neck].

A lack of blood swipes on the door and blood drops on the floor
leading into the communion preparation room where the
victim was found indicates that the fatal assault occurred in the
preparation room rather than in the main chapel.

There were no visible vertical blood drops or smears on the floor tiles,
walls, or furniture within the preparation room. This lack of blood
suggests that the victim was attacked and rendered unconscious or
immobile quickly. The blood spatter patterns that are visible on
the victim and her clothing, as well as some medium-velocity
blood spatter on the floor adjacent to her head, are consistent with
the stabbing having occurred with the victim on the floor.

It is apparent that the position or orientation of the altar cloth and
victim's clothing were not consistent throughout the entire
stabbing event. The initial set of stabbings occurred with a portion of the altar cloth on her left chest, covering wound sites.
The wounds associated with some of these initial stabbings
were very minor. Those minor wounds barely penetrated the
skin and had very little bleeding associated with them. These
wounds were in a pattern formation. The pattern is consistent
with a cross shape. This pattern of stab wounds is not a typical
type of stabbing death.

After the altar cloth was removed from the victim's chest region,
additional stabbings occurred. Most of these additional stab
wounds were deep and had extensive bleeding associated with
them. These wounds are commonly associated with a frenzied
type of killing.

Examination of the various layers of the victim's clothing indicates
that many of the stab holes are aligned, thus indicating a relative lack of movement from the victim during much of the

stabbing, which likely occurred once the victim was disabled and lying on the floor. The outer blue dress was most likely pushed upward by the suspect as indicated by the presence of blood spatters on the upper inner surfaces of the dress.

Microscopic examination of the victim's clothing and altar cloth indicated that the defects or holes were consistent with a sharp instrument, but not a typical flat, straight-bladed knife. The unique shape of these cuts is consistent with having been created by a curved sharp blade such as the letter opener blade.

Application of TMB, a bloody print enhancement reagent, to the altar cloth revealed a blood contact transfer pattern with a general pattern and circular configuration similar to the medallion portion of the letter opener. A further macroscopic and microscopic examination was suggested to investigators for a more detailed comparison.

Based on the original crime scene photographs, autopsy results, laboratory analysis, and subsequent examinations, the death of Sister Pahl occurred in the small preparation room, adjacent to the main chapel. She was first taken by surprise, then disabled on the floor. A sexual attack or attempt likely occurred as indicated by her dress being pushed upward. Subsequently, additional stabbing occurred. Initial stab wounds were more likely on her left chest area with the altar cloth covering this area of her chest or even her face. A sharp, narrow blade-type of instrument was used. A cross-shape type of wound pattern was inflicted. Thereafter, the altar cloth was removed and more stab wounds were inflicted while the victim was on the floor.

Dr. Henry C. Lee:

There are five different types of sharp instrument wounds: stab, cut, chip, slash, and scrape. In a stab wound, its measured depth is greater than its length. Stab wounds are at the forensic core of this case.

Thus it is fitting to consider the following, while keeping in mind that stab wounds may be homicidal, suicidal, or accidental. We shall restrict our comments to those involved in a homicidal act.

Usually these types of wounds are produced by sharp, pointed instruments such as knives, screwdrivers, ice picks, or open scissors, but sometimes a blunter instrument, such as a poker or a closed pair of scissors, is responsible. As a general rule, the blunter the instrument, the more ragged the entry hole and the more bruised the surrounding skin. There are exceptions, however, as in the case of a victim's twisting around or the assailant's turning the weapon in the wound. Both these maneuvers can have an impact on any estimation of the weapon's width and therefore interfere with its possible identification.

The most common weapon is a knife, and its entry hole might be in the form of a slit, especially if the knife is double-edged, like a dagger. In contrast, a single-edged knife leaves a hole that tapers at one end. As in a case like Phil Spector's (see chapter 1), where the angle of a gunshot wound and the deposition pattern of gunshot residue might help determine the location from which the gun was fired, so too can knife wound characteristics give a clue to the way the knife was used. For example, a jab or thrusting motion at a right angle to the target surface might be expected to produce a deep puncture wound, whereas a slashing motion would inflict a long but superficial cut. In the case of multiple wounds, a keen forensic pathologist may even be able to reconstruct the timing of the stabbings and to determine which of them actually caused the most damage or was, in fact, the fatal wound.

If a knife is recovered, important forensic information might be gained by simple but careful inspection of it. It can retain blood belonging to the victim, and possibly to the assailant, thereby rendering such findings as blood groupings and DNA. And, of course, fingerprints could be developed.

Stab wounds involve an external (skin) component and an internal (deeper) component. As the expert forensic pathologist Dr. Vincent Di Maio points out:

- A distinguishing characteristic of stab wounds is the absence of "bridging tissue" in the depth of the wound. If connecting tissue strands are present in the base of the wound, it is more likely the wound was produced by a blow with a blunt object, and not a stab with a sharp-edged implement, as the latter would cut through, not tear the tissue. Therefore, the terms **laceration** and **stab wound** (or **cut**) should never be used interchangeably.
- Other terms associated with stab wounds include **puncture**, **penetrating**, and **perforating**. A **puncture** wound is the piercing of the body by a sharp-tipped object. It tends to have more depth than width, which distinguishes it from a cut. Once the weapon has passed through the victim's clothes, the body offers little resistance unless the weapon encounters bone (which was the case with Sister Pahl, as we shall soon see during trial testimony).
- Wounds that enter an organ are referred to as **penetrating** wounds, and if they also pass out the other side they are known as **perforating** wounds. Virtually any stab wound may produce internal bleeding—sometimes massive—even if its external appearance seems trivial.
- From a forensic standpoint, it is not simply the nature of the wounds on and in a victim that matters; it is also their pattern. (Sometimes the pattern conveys a message but the presence of nine chest stabbings in the shape of an inverted cross,

as in this case, is a rare occurrence.) Contusions [bruises] and lacerations widely scattered over the arms, legs, and torso may be indicative of struggle or torture. **Defensive** stab wounds appear usually on the hands, the back aspects of the forearms, or backs of the upper arms of the victim. They are produced when the victim tries to defend himself/herself from the assailant.[32]

DI MAIO CONTINUES:

A patterned skin abrasion or contusion may be produced by the guard of the knife contacting the skin if the weapon is driven into the body with great force. The guard on a knife is a separate piece of metal which is perpendicularly attached to the blade, between the blade and the handle, which keeps the hand away from the blade while cutting. . . . Single-edged weapons may produce skin wounds in which both ends are squared off or blunted, if the weapon has been driven in up to the guard. This happens because in most knives, a short section of the blade (ricasso) immediately in front of the guard is unsharpened on both edges. . . . If the knife or stabbing weapon encounters bone, the tip of the weapon may break off and remain in the body. For this reason, victims stabbed multiple times, or having stab wounds into bone, should be radiographed prior to autopsy.

> . . . [In] homicidal stabbings:
> - multiple wounds are usually present, with most penetrating deep into the body;
> - most fatal chest wounds involve injury to the heart or aorta. A stab wound to the heart that severs the left anterior descending artery can cause rapid death;

- the abdominal organs may be injured by stab wounds to the abdomen or lower chest; fatal stab wounds of the abdomen usually involve the liver and/or a major blood vessel. Abdominal stab wounds may cause delayed death due to peritonitis [infection involving the membrane lining the abdominal cavity], and sepsis [generalized invasion of the body by microorganisms or their toxins];
- wounds of the head and neck are less common than wounds to the chest and abdomen.

Stab wounds of the neck cause death acutely by exsanguinations [drainage of blood], air embolism, or asphyxia by compression of the neck organs if massive soft tissue hemorrhage is present.

Delayed death may occur from cellulitis [inflammation of cellular tissue such as skin, muscle, or other soft tissue] or arterial thrombosis [blood clotting] leading to cerebral infarction [tissue death].

If stab wounds are present in the neck, a postmortem radiograph of the chest should be made prior to autopsy, as an aid in demonstrating air embolism.

Fatal stab wounds of the head are uncommon. When present, they may cause injury to the skull or brain.[33]

THE TRIAL

Jurors in the three-week-long trial heard testimony from a total of forty-one witnesses, thirty for the prosecution and eleven for the defense. Each day, Judge Thomas Osowik's wood-paneled second-floor courtroom was filled to capacity.

In opening statements on Friday, April 21, 2006, Dean Mandros, assistant Lucas County prosecutor, told the panel that he would not be presenting them with a motive because under the law, the prosecution did not have to prove motive in order to prove murder. But he did indicate it would prove that a sword-shaped letter opener belonging to the defendant was used in the brutal murder the day before Easter in 1980. He stated that the unusual shape of the blade fit the victim's wounds "like a key in a lock." Mandros further claimed that Father Robinson had lied about his whereabouts on the morning of the murder and that he would produce witnesses who could place Robinson at the chapel at the time of the slaying. And there were other lies, he said.

"The defendant made statements that were just plainly not true," he declared, looking straight at the priest, whose eyes were closed as if sleeping. "He denied ever having a key to the sacristy. He even claimed that someone else had confessed to doing the killing to him. And when pressed on the matter, he admitted, no, he'd made that up. That wasn't true at all."

The prosecutor outlined details of the crime in a thorough, professional, and scientific manner while Father Robinson, wearing his priest's collar, continued to register no emotion.

Mandros said, "She [Sister Margaret Ann] was working on the altar and it was in the sacristy of that chapel [where] someone took her by the neck and choked her so hard that a [bone] broke on the side of her neck. Blood vessels in her eyes burst as she was choked to the verge of death."

Father Robinson laid her on the floor of the sacristy, Mandros continued, then draped her body with an altar cloth and proceeded to stab her nine times over the heart in the shape of an upside-down cross. The prosecutor stated that the defendant next stabbed her twenty-two more times before pulling up her skirt and lowering her undergarments to leave her lying half-naked on the floor. There was no evidence of sexual assault, he said, and authorities quickly concluded that the killing was the work of someone the victim knew.

"Strangers don't typically have that type of energy, emotional anger, to stab someone thirty-one times."[34]

Meanwhile, defense attorney Alan Konop likened the state's case to an incomplete jigsaw puzzle, saying the evidence against his client was just as scarce now as it had been back in 1980. He stressed the fact that the state's evidence was purely circumstantial and contained flaws that raised reasonable doubts. He indicated, for example, that DNA tests of a foreign substance on the nun's undergarment did not match that of Father Robinson, and that material found under her fingernails contained a male chromosome that did not match the priest's.

"In 1980, when the original investigation began, you will find from witnesses that there were important inconsistencies and discrepancies," the defense attorney said. "You'll also find some old witnesses from 1980 that gave a new spin in 2003, that added some information twenty-three or twenty-four years after the event."

He told the panel that Father Robinson, now sixty-eight and a long-time suspect in the case, was arrested before any reports or testing were done. Even after Sister Margaret Ann's body was exhumed for DNA testing, he said authorities were still unable to link his client to the murder.

"There's an indictment and arrest first, and then the questions are asked," he alleged. "This is all being done after the humiliation and degradation of an arrest of Father Robinson."[35]

Witnesses for the Prosecution

Most of the major witnesses for each side were individuals we've already discussed.

The first two for the prosecution were seventy-nine-year-old Sister Phyllis Ann Gerold, the former CEO of Mercy Hospital, and Sister Madelyn Marie Gordon, its chapel organist.

Sister Phyllis Ann spoke of racing from the dining room to the chapel upon hearing the piercing screams of Sister Madelyn Marie; of seeing Sister Margaret Ann dead on the floor of the sacristy; and, with the use of a mannequin, described the position of the body and the location of the victim's clothes.

Mandros asked her to describe her first impression upon seeing the body and then to elaborate on its position. The nun responded: "The horror. I think it was the weirdness of it and that she needed to be saved.

And then the afterthought 'Why the ritualistic kind of layout of a dead body?'" She spoke softly but deliberately. "I remember [its position] was so neat and so different. I told them it was ritualistic. She was lying in the center on the floor and I saw no blood. If I remember correctly, her arms were straight. Her legs were straight. And all her clothes from probably her brassiere all the way down [were] rolled down to her feet. People don't usually die very straight."[36]

Sister Madelyn Marie, now in her eighties, was then called to the stand; she was the one who had found the dead body. She characterized Sister Margaret Ann as a perfectionist and then gave an explicit account of the discovery. Her emotional testimony transfixed the jury as she struggled to find words for her version of the body's position. As it turned out, her version was a near duplicate of Sister Phyllis Ann's.

Other witnesses during the first six days of testimony were two detectives, one coroner, six forensic experts, two housekeepers, a hospital janitor, and an authority on the occult. Most offered information that we have referenced before, but we shall now highlight the testimony of six of them.

Terry Cousino of the Toledo Police Department's Scientific Investigations Unit was the first of them to testify. Testimony by the widely experienced crime scene investigator lasted two hours. Utilizing a large display screen, he called attention to distinctive bloodstains that closely resembled the highly unusual letter opener. At one point, he referred to the knob at the upper end of the blade as shaped like an acorn, and to certain linear patterns as mimicking the ridges in the handle.

With Judge Osowik's permission, the ten-foot-long altar cloth was then laid out on the floor before the jury box, and jurors were invited to walk around it for closer inspection of the residual stains and numerous stab holes. Cousino described the pattern of the holes in detail.

"There are eighteen," he explained, "and they're pretty much centered in the altar cloth."

He said it did not take long for him to realize the cloth had been folded in half, thus resulting in nine holes lining up perfectly and forming an inverted cross.

"[It] jumps out at you," he told the jury. "Not only did it fit the form of a cross, the symmetry and the precision of it would suggest to me that something was used as a template to put down on the cloth and stab around."

Cousino next turned to the letter opener, describing it as highly unusual in appearance and in construction, with its diamond-shaped blade and medallion. He suggested that the blade and the holes matched, while describing the holes as "highly unusual."

"I've seen many different stab defects in clothing," he stated, "but I have never seen ones like that. They're normally just a slit. Even if it's a wider blade, it usually looks like a fat slit. But this 'Y' shape was very unique."[37]

Deputy Coroner Dr. Diane Scala-Barnett testified that she had performed approximately seven thousand autopsies in her career and that she was the successor to Dr. Renate Fazekas, the pathologist who had conducted the victim's original autopsy. Scala-Barnett told the jury that Sister Margaret Ann had probably been choked from the back with a soft ligature like a cloth, because her necklace and cross, inscribed "I AM A CATHOLIC. PLEASE CALL A PRIEST," had made an impression in her skin.

"That could be consistent with a soft ligature strangulation," she said, "because it's not leaving any other marks."

She then elaborated on how the hyoid bone in the neck might become fractured during a strangulation, and why—based on her predecessor's notations about the wounds—she believed scissors could not have been the murder weapon.

"Are there any indications that she was alive and moving when she was being stabbed?" the prosecution asked.

"There was no indication of any movement," the pathologist replied. "If a person was alive and moving...you'd expect defense wounds. If a person is conscious...fighting. Shielding themselves, or trying to grab the weapon."

"Were any defense wounds noted?"

"None."

Then the doctor described the autopsy on the victim's remains in 2004, after her body had been exhumed. "Believe it or not," she said to the jury, "twenty-four years later, you could still see many of the stab wounds in the actual skin and in the soft tissue."

She went on to say that besides taking DNA samples, she had removed pieces of bone, including the mandible (lower jaw). Later, together with forensic anthropologist Julie Saul, she tested to see if the letter opener fit into a "small diamond-shaped defect" found in the mandible.

"It was a perfect fit," she declared.

"Based on your testing," the prosecution inquired, "did you draw a conclusion, based on a reasonable degree of scientific or medical certainty, as to what caused this injury to this mandible?"

"It was my conclusion," said the deputy coroner, "based on my experience, my knowledge, my training, that this weapon [the letter opener] caused these injuries, or a weapon exactly like this."[38]

As expected, leading bloodstain pattern expert T. Paulette Sutton focused on that subject during her testimony. With the aid of photographs, charts, and diagrams, she demonstrated various transfer patterns and how they related to the letter opener. Specifically, she laid a transparency of the letter opener's medallion over a stain on the altar cloth, showing where the bloody lines defined the domed roof of the US Capitol building. In addition, she pointed out a semicircular stain on the victim's forehead that matched another part of the opener, asserting that the killer had no doubt pressed the bloody handle into Sister Margaret Ann's forehead.

On cross-examination, the defense suggested that Sutton's findings were skewed because prosecutors gave her only one possible weapon, the letter opener, for comparison. The defense lawyer had the witness trace a pair of scissors and hold them up to the mark she had identified as consistent with the opener.

"It could be a pair of scissors, yes," she said. And in fact a pair of scissors was found to be missing from the chapel after the murder. But when the prosecution asked if she had ever seen a pair of scissors with the Washington skyline on them, she answered that she had not.[39]

I was called to the stand on the fifth day of the trial and testified for about forty-five minutes. I remember prosecutor Christopher Anderson asking me to inspect some black and white photographs of the crime scene, at which point I took out my trusty magnifying glass from my briefcase.

"Doctor," he asked, "do you always carry a magnifying glass?"

"I always carry one," I replied. "It's my basic tool. You don't know when you're going to be called to a crime scene to examine evidence, and you can't carry a microscope around." The jury members chuckled.

Displaying photographs of the altar cloth bloodstains on a large flat screen when testifying, I directed attention to similarities between transfer patterns and the letter opener, and told the jury that certain elements of an image in one stain could be attributed to the Capitol building medallion on the letter opener. This would hold, I said, especially after the application of a bloodstain enhancement reagent that would make the pattern stand out.

"It is consistent," I said. "I cannot come here to tell you this pattern is produced exactly by this. I can only say 'similar to.' I emphasized that it couldn't be excluded."

I gave my opinion that Sister Margaret Ann was murdered in a quick attack and probably strangled before being stabbed. "She was not standing up ... for if that were the case, we should see vertical blood drops running down."

In his testimony, Dr. Steven Symes, another renowned forensic anthropologist with a special expertise in knife wounds on bone, illustrated how the diamond or star-shaped wounds on the victim's body matched the shape of the letter opener.

And finally, Father Jeffrey Grob, associate canonical vicar for the Archdiocese of Chicago and an expert in exorcism and other Roman Catholic rituals, testified that the murder was committed by someone with specialized knowledge of the church's rites and symbols—namely, a member of the clergy. He explained that the circumstances of the killing, including the use of an altar cloth and an apparent anointing of Sister Margaret Ann in blood, indicated a more thorough understanding of the faith than lay Catholics possess.

The prosecutor asked him to point out some ritualistic aspects of the crime.

"Where does one begin?" the priest sighed. He said that in the eyes of the church, a nun is a virgin wed to God, and that by leaving Sister Margaret Ann naked, the killer was "defiling the bride of Christ." He declared that profaning that which is holy and pure is a hallmark of satanic worship.

"You take innocence and you destroy or mock it," he said.

Grob further explained that the upside-down cross was used in satanic ceremonies as an "affront to the sacred," and that the use of the cloth showed a desire to "penetrate" the holy with the evil. He believed the bloody semicircle on the nun's forehead might be evidence that the murderer performed a perverse version of the sacrament of last rites—a Catholic ritual in which the head and hands of a dying or gravely ill person are anointed with oil—on Sister Margaret Ann.

"It's a reversal," he said. "Normally, what should be a good Catholic person going to meet God, getting anointed, is now all of a sudden mocking. [She is] anointed with blood, her own blood."[40]

Key prosecution witnesses in the second week of the trial called to the stand to place Father Robinson near the chapel around the time of the murder included Leslie Kerner, a former EKG technician; Grace Jones, a former laboratory worker; and Dr. Jack Baron, chief resident at the hospital at the time of the murder.

The state's final witness, Detective Tom Ross, informed the jury of several inconsistencies between what the defendant had told the police and what was contained in his taped interrogation. The detective played selections of the tape to illustrate his claims.

Mandros then rested the state's case. Strangely, over seven full days of testimony, the prosecution had called a total of thirty-one witnesses—the same as the number of stab wounds inflicted on the victim.

Witnesses for the Defense

The defense called only eleven witnesses, about a third as many as the prosecution. The first was Detective Steve Forrester, who was summoned in an attempt to discredit the three former hospital employees' damning testimony about the defendant's whereabouts during the time of the crime. Most of the remaining defense witnesses were former police officers, a ploy that played right into the hands of the prosecution. Mandros would later explain that he had made a strategic decision not to call many of the original 1980 detectives. It proved to be a brilliant move.

"We felt that if we didn't call them, the defense would. And that would give us an advantage. For when I call a witness, I can only use direct questioning and not any leading questions. But if they call a witness, when I cross-examine them, I can use leading questions. So I can control the testimony a thousand times more. The cross-examination is, in effect, the lawyer's opportunity to testify," said Mandros, who happens to teach trial law.[41]

The strategy paid off during testimony by detectives Forrester, Marx, and Vetter. In the cross-examination of each of them, the prosecution appeared to score points.

Even testimony by Dr. Kathleen Reichs seemed to backfire. Billed as the defense's star witness, she is a nationally recognized forensic anthropologist, a best-selling crime author, and the inspiration for the hit TV series *Bones*. She is also a friend of mine.

She stated that she had studied all of the following: the 1980s police reports, Dr. Fazeka's original autopsy report, Dr. Scala-Barnett's exhumation report, the skeletal analysis of Drs. Julie and Frank Saul, and also photographs of the victim's mandible and other bones. Defense attorney John Thebes then asked her professional opinion about placing the tip of the letter opener into Sister Margaret Ann's mandible.

"In my opinion," said Reichs, "you would never do that, because of the potential for damage or modification of the defect."

"You did not look at that mandible itself?" Thebes asked. "Why?"

"Given that something was inserted into it at least once," Reichs replied, "any analysis subsequent to that becomes compromised. You don't know if damage was done at the time that the object was stuck in there. So for me to look at it would be irrelevant."

A betting person would say that Anderson couldn't wait to cross-examine. He asked the anthropologist if she had actually examined any of the evidence firsthand. She admitted she had not.

"Is it normally a protocol for anthropology," Anderson inquired, "if you're given a problem, you define it, and then you take steps towards analyzing it or coming up with a solution?"

"Yes," she replied.

"And normally that involves viewing or handling the actual material?"

"Most cases," Reichs answered. "Not all cases. Sometimes you might work from images."

"How many times have you testified in court strictly from images?"

"I've never testified strictly from images," she said.

"This is the first one?" Anderson asked, scanning the jury.

"I'm testifying here on protocol and methodology," she stated.

"You're not testifying as to the results?"

"No."

Score more points for the prosecution as the defense rested its case.[42]

Closing Arguments

Both closing arguments contained little that was new, certainly nothing startling. Mandros told the jury that although prosecutors are not required to prove motive, he held that Father Robinson lashed out at strong-willed Sister Margaret Ann because of mounting disagreements, because of his having been passed over for a position as a military chaplain, and because he really loathed his responsibilities in giving last rites and comforting the sick.

"He had enough," Mandros maintained. "The man decided he had enough. He had taken a lot, but he wasn't going to take it anymore."

For whatever reason—probably tactical from a legal point of view—the lawyer minimized the idea that the nun was killed as an offering of human sacrifice to a diabolical power.

"Is this some kind of satanic cult killing? No. Is this some ritualistic Black Mass? No, sorry to disappoint," he said. "This case is about perhaps the most common scenario there is for homicide: A man got very angry at a woman and the woman died. The only thing different is that the man wore a white collar and the woman wore a habit."

Mandros stated that the inverted cross, the exposing of the nun's genitals, and an apparent anointing of her forehead with blood were "a bastardized version" of the last rites the priest hated to perform and were designed, he said, his voice rising, "to degrade her, to mock her, to humiliate her, to bring her down to the lowest point he possibly could."[43]

He then referred to time and change. "Some things don't really change with the passage of time," he said. "And the heart of the State's case is just the same now as it was on April fifth, 1980. The letter opener is just the same now as it was back in April 1980, when it was put in that police property room, where it stayed for some twenty-four years. This altar cloth, these stains are just the same."

The lead prosecutor next delved into a review of the physical evidence, Robinson's physical accountability around the time of the slaying, and his false confession.

"Now we don't expect priests to kill, do we?" he asked. "But do we expect them to lie to the police during a murder investigation? Who lies to the police during a murder investigation? Maybe the one [who] did the crime."

Mandros then addressed Father Robinson's state of mind in more detail, defining the priest's 1980 world as one limited to "darkness and death."

The bulk of the closing dealt with the prosecution's step-by-step theory of what transpired on that Holy Saturday morning in 1980.

Then, turning toward the defense table where an impassive Father Robinson sat, Mandros told the jury: "And if that white collar means anything to him, he has always known that one day he is going to be held accountable for what he has done. So for all these years, he's been waiting. And now he's waiting for you."[44]

The defense's closing was delivered in two parts, one by Konop and one by Thebes. Straight away, Thebes said that Father Robinson was not guilty because the state had not proven beyond a reasonable doubt that the letter opener was the murder weapon. He claimed its entire prosecution was predicated on such an assumption. The substance of his next forty minutes of summation consisted of dismissing all the prosecution's expert witness testimony, claiming the findings were invalid because they were not objective.

"This forensic evidence takes many forms," he said, pacing before the jury box. "I think you could group it into four basic areas. We had blood transfer. We had forensic pathology. We had forensic anthropology—the bones—and we had DNA....Every [state] expert called was an expert in a subjective field. They rely on experts in those fields of subjectivity."

Thebes next insisted that the murder weapon was the missing pair of scissors. He reminded the jury that the late Dr. Renate Fazekas had found the stab wounds consistent with being caused by scissors. "But Dr. Scala-Barnett," Thebes said, "who is part of the cold case team, contradicts her mentor and said it had to be the dagger."

Then the defender contradicted his own earlier claim that DNA should be included in a group of subjective fields. He told the jury that DNA evidence *is* objective, but that after results had demonstrated none of Father Robinson's on the victim's underclothing, the state had "turned a blind eye."

Konop's share of the closing lasted eighty minutes, during which time he focused on (1) his contention that the state's case was entirely circumstantial and (2) tearing apart the 1980 investigation. He said that the murder scene had not been processed properly and that no fingerprints and only a few trace evidence samples were obtained. He accused the state of being so short on evidence, they had to play the Catholic card.

"They must be pretty darn desperate to have to blame it on the Church," he stated. "Maybe they should blame it on their own investigation."

Konop concluded his remarks before an increasingly restless jury with: "[Now it's your turn] to render a verdict so that when you see Father Robinson with his friends and family, you can go up to him and say, 'Father Robinson, I was on the jury that did the right thing. And the right thing was this—the State didn't have a case beyond a reasonable doubt, and we stood up for the law. We enforced the law to find you not guilty by law.'"[45]

THE VERDICT

It took the jury only six-and-a-half hours of deliberation to find Father Robinson guilty, marking the first time in American history that a Catholic priest was convicted of murdering a nun. Osowik immediately sentenced him to the mandatory term of fifteen years to life in prison. The priest did not visibly react to the verdict, but his family and friends gasped when it was read. A courtroom deputy handcuffed Robinson, now a convicted murderer, and led him away.

Later, Leonard Blair, bishop of the Diocese of Toledo, issued an official statement. It read: "Let us hope that the conclusion of the trial will bring some measure of healing for all those affected by the case as well as for our local church. The diocese has remained steadfast in the work of the Church and its ministries throughout this trial, and will continue to do so."[46]

POSTSCRIPT

This was a case of many "possibles": a personality feud that possibly turned deadly, a possible satanic murder, a possible cover-up by the Catholic Diocese of Toledo, possible collusion involving elements of the Toledo Police Department, and possible eyewitness identification. But it was also a case that provided a close look at how a decades-old murder case could eventually be resurrected and solved, at how the perseverance of law enforcement officials can be tested, and at how forensic science and its practitioners can work their magic.

As for the trial, some observers felt its most dramatic moment came when Mandros played parts of a video of Father Robinson's interview with police just after he was arrested. Left alone for a few minutes and unaware he was still being videotaped, the priest appeared close to tears as he lowered his head and whispered, "Oh, my Jesus. Sister, won't you come through for me? Please. Won't you?"[47]

Makes you wonder, doesn't it?

4

A Police Shooting and the Public Trust

Among the hazards most police officers face are (a) being shot in the line of duty, (b) accidentally shooting a suspect, and (c) having to shoot a suspect the officer believes is about to fire at him. The last situation is at the heart of the following case. The shooting took place in Hartford, Connecticut, on April 13, 1999. I was the state's commissioner of public safety at the time.

SUMMARY OF THE CASE

"Am I going to die?"

These may have been the last words of fourteen-year-old Aquan Salmon, according to his friend, Ellis Thomas, age fifteen. Salmon had been shot by Hartford police officer Robert Allan. The teenagers, along with two others, were robbery suspects—occupants in a white Cadillac that Allan was following in his cruiser. After Salmon's death, the other three—Thomas; Dennis Faniel, age fourteen; and Robert Davis III, age fifteen—were charged with first-degree robbery and second-degree assault in connection with the mugging and pistol-whipping of a Hartford woman. Salmon, Thomas, Faniel, and Davis—all African Americans—had been pursued by Allan, who is white.

At least two different accounts emerged of what took place early April 13 in a dark vacant lot in Hartford's north end. One account came from Thomas and the other was from Officer Allan (see pages 184–87). According to Thomas, he and his three friends bolted because Allan was chasing them in his patrol car. He said they had rented the Cadillac— which had been reported stolen in New Britain, Connecticut, earlier that evening—for fifteen dollars and Thomas was the driver. He turned into the lot on Enfield Street shortly after 2:00 a.m., followed by Allan in his cruiser. Thomas was the first to run from the car. He stated he then climbed over a chain-link fence and watched the shooting from his hiding spot. Faniel scrambled from the car and made it to a friend's house nearby. Salmon exited the car next, and Davis remained inside. It was at this point that Thomas's statement differs from the police officer's.

"As I was running, I didn't have anything in my hands, and Aquan didn't either," Thomas told state police investigators. "The cop was chasing us. He didn't say anything to us. I had jumped over the fence. The cop then said he was going to shoot, and Aquan put his hands up over his head. Aquan tried to turn around but the cop didn't let him because he shot him.... When Aquan got hit, the bullet spinned him around." Thomas said Allan went to his car and reported the shooting on his radio. He returned to Salmon with another police officer and "[that's when] Aquan asked if he going to die and the cop told him he was going to be all right," Thomas said.[1]

Police called for an ambulance and Salmon was taken to a local hospital's emergency room, where he was pronounced dead. The reported manner of death was a single gunshot in the back of his left shoulder blade.

Allan, on the other hand, stated he had his flashlight in one hand and his gun in the other when he emerged from his vehicle. He claimed he heard what he thought was a gunshot and saw someone running toward him from the right. He said the person ignored his order to freeze and the person appeared to be reaching toward his belt. Allan reported he feared for his life when he fired the shot. An authentic-looking toy gun and handgun-shaped cigarette lighter were later found at the scene.

PUBLIC REACTION

Public reaction was swift—some of it angry, some tolerant, most of it measured. It was not long after the incident that the black community—in Connecticut's capital city and beyond—specifically articulated the perception that Salmon had been shot in the back, and that it was therefore an execution-style shooting. Some black leaders were restrained in their response, recommending measures that would help young people to avoid trouble, but also ones that would provide cultural sensitivity training to police cadets by requiring them to live temporarily in black or Hispanic neighborhoods. Others were more critical, recalling a similar incident concerning an African American Connecticut man just four months before, when twenty-seven-year-old Franklyn Reid had been killed by Officer Scott Smith in New Milford, a town in northwestern Connecticut near the New York State line. Still others used the tragedy as a rallying point to advance the cause of civil rights.

"People of color are losing their lives at the hands of white police officers," said Reverend Nora Wyatt Jr. of the Greater Hartford African American Alliance. "It's not a lot of white people losing their lives."[2]

State Representative Marie Kirkley-Bey called for stricter guidelines for police on when they can use deadly force. "No one has the right to take someone's life on a thought," she said.[3]

It quickly became obvious to politicians, law enforcement officials, and the public at large that racial tensions were simmering in certain quarters and had risen to a fever pitch in others. Some observers expressed fear of an eventual incendiary outcome: race riots.

A public hearing was held at Hartford's Legislative Office Building before the governor's Law Enforcement Council. The council was seeking comments on how to improve and standardize investigations of police shootings. During the hearing, I testified and then issued a public statement indicating that Salmon was not shot in the back, that the police officer's bullet entered the side of Salmon's shoulder blade, three and a half inches from his spine, and exited through the right chest. (In other words, the bullet came at Salmon at an oblique angle.) Foremost on my mind was the sensitive nature of the case, and I wanted to stress that it was important to know that it was not simply a shooting where the bullet entered the back and exited from the front (in a straight line). I stated that it was just as important to know that (a) the bullet trajectory went from the *left* back to the *right* front and (b) the autopsy report noted a trajectory of 45 degrees, indicating only the impact angle, not the direction. The angle of the shot suggested that Allan was not directly behind the youth but to the side of him when he fired.

In any event, I was asked to conduct a crime scene reconstruction for New London State's Attorney Kevin Kane, who would later decide whether or not Allan acted lawfully. In a written statement, Governor John Rowland had ordered the investigation to be taken out of the hands of the Hartford Police Department. Jack Bailey, the chief state's attorney, complied, appointing Kane as a special prosecutor in charge of the investigation. Rowland had drawn on a newly enacted statute permitting such a move to avoid a possible conflict of interest in cases involving the use of deadly force by police.

He wrote: "Without passing judgment on the officer's actions, I believe it is in the best interest of the citizens of Hartford and the city's police department to ensure this investigation is conducted by an outside and impartial law enforcement agency."[4]

The statute itself (commonly referred to as the "Deadly Force Law") says, in part, that a police officer

> is justified in using deadly physical force upon another person only when he reasonably believes such is necessary to: (1) defend himself or a third person from the use or imminent use of deadly force; or (2) effect an arrest or prevent the escape from custody of a person [who] he reasonably believes has committed or has attempted to commit a felony which involved the infliction or threatened infliction of serious physical injury and if, where feasible, he has given warning of his intent to use deadly physical force.[5]

Of Kane's new role, Michael Buerger, a criminal justice professor at Northeastern University who was considered an authority in shootings involving police, said, "Prosecutors are human. And, in some instances, political ramifications and how a case would play before a jury have played a role, but typically they are not major factors."

The professor, a former New Hampshire police officer, added, "Still, the questions are: Was there clear and present danger, and was there an identifiable threat?"[6]

At about the same time, black and Latino residents gathered at a Hartford church and charged that the shooting was symptomatic of deep-seated problems in the police department. They asked Kane and his associates to recall a 1973 federal court decree that set guidelines for training, supervision, and the use of deadly force in the department. The decree settled a class-action lawsuit concerning the fatal shooting of a nineteen-year-old Latino man by a Hartford police officer in 1969.

"Had that decree been followed faithfully, Aquan Salmon would be alive today," asserted Joseph Moniz, a prominent criminal defense attorney who represented the family of Malik Jones, the victim of another police shooting two years earlier in the New Haven area. Moniz was asked by Puerto Rican and other community organizations to see whether or not Hartford had violated the terms of the decree. But he went a step further, urging Kane to consider language in the decree that goes beyond Connecticut's deadly force statutes—in effect adding a layer of protection against police shootings for those who are sixteen years of age and under.

However, Sergeant Michael Wood, head of the Hartford police union, strongly objected. "The thing is," he said, "how was Robert Allan going to know in the dark, with his attention trained on another suspect, that the person coming at him was under sixteen?"

And state lawmaker Michael Lawlor, chairman of the judiciary committee and a former prosecutor, dismissed the relevance of the 1973 decree out of hand. "Kevin Kane's only responsibility is to determine whether the shooting is justified under Connecticut law," he said. He added that the US Department of Justice could possibly decide to initiate a civil rights action, but he emphasized that the consent decree "does not supersede the state's law on deadly force."

Most opinion makers agreed that Kane's primary responsibility was to decide if Allan's action stemmed from a reasonable belief that his life was in jeopardy. In this regard, some cited New Haven State's Attorney Michael Dearington, who cleared the police officer in the Malik Jones case, noting in his report that the US Supreme Court judged reasonableness "from the perspective of a reasonable officer at the scene, rather than with the 20/20 vision of hindsight."[7]

Others invoked a 1989 case in which the same high court ruled that the "calculus for reasonableness [must allow for the fact that] police officers are often forced to make split-second judgments—in circumstances that are tense, uncertain and rapidly evolving—about the amount of force necessary in a particular situation."[8]

As can be seen in this discussion, there are special issues that arise in the cases of shootings by police officers. If these cases are not investigated and handled correctly, the involved police agency, individual officer(s), and entire criminal justice system will likely face severe criticism, loss of public trust and confidence, and exposure to extensive civil liability. Police chiefs, district attorneys, and government leaders need to prepare for the high level of scrutiny that such an incident and their subsequent actions should and will undergo. Additionally, they must formulate their plans in a manner that guarantees as much independent objectivity into the investigation as possible. Furthermore, they must recognize difficulties that often complicate "police-involved shootings," such as lack of witnesses.

Police shootings certainly attract significant media attention and public interest. Public impressions are often established in the early hours of the investigation, even with little or no input from the police department. It is therefore imperative to report relevant information to the media through an organized public information system—and this must be done expeditiously and accurately. Sometimes a single spokesperson from the police agency is sufficient to interact with news reporters. Failure to respond to basic media inquiries will likely be viewed as a defensive posture. However, caution must be exercised not to be premature in making comments or drawing conclusions. As the investigation proceeds to its conclusion, it is often beneficial for the investigators to meet with civic leaders and groups, with media representatives, with family members, and with legal counsel for both the involved police officer(s) and the shooting victim's family.

Since perceptions take on a reality of their own, police chiefs and leaders must keep this in mind as they proceed. Wherever possible, the entire investigation should be conducted by an external agency. The district attorney will have the ultimate responsibility for determining whether or not the shooting was lawful and justified. However, police or laboratory personnel will likely conduct the crime scene processing and investigation. If there are insufficient local resources for an outside agency to provide the crime scene and investigative functions, then supervisors need to ensure that all personnel taking part in the investigation are not closely associated with any of the involved officers. The issue here, of course, is conflict of interest. And since the case will no doubt be highly probed and litigated in some forum—such as a civil court—every available resource and expert should be utilized. If the forensic laboratory or crime scene unit has experts in shooting reconstruction or related disciplines, it would be advantageous to involve them as soon as possible, ideally at the initial crime scene.

There are some common characteristics involved in police shootings that can create special challenges. In many cases, there is, as noted earlier, a lack of witnesses—or at least **available** witnesses—during the early portion of the investigation. Sometimes those who do come forward may be biased toward the victim or the police officer(s). At other times, the individual wounded during the encounter may be dead or incapacitated to the point where an interview is deemed impossible. In cases where the shooter's racial background differs from that of the victim (as occurred in the Hartford case), certain sensitivity issues must be confronted head-on and discreetly managed. Prompt attention to these factors will go a long way in keeping local racial relations from becoming unglued.

The officers involved in the shooting frequently choose to exercise their constitutionally protected rights and make themselves available for questioning at a later date in the presence of legal counsel. As a result, it is possible that the crime scene unit will need to perform their functions with little or no background information. But that background is not initially crucial: All crime scene photographs, autopsy reports and photographs, videotapes of the scene, measurements, notes, crime scene reports, and laboratory reports of physical evidence testing will be processed and then must be judiciously studied. Whenever possible—as in the case of **any** shooting—early direct observation of the crime scene and the collection of relevant evidence are most desirable. Complete and accurate documentation is absolutely essential. Direct examination of the physical evidence to detect any type of damage, stains, and related conditions will provide the best opportunity for later reconstruction analysis. It should be noted that complete reconstructions are often not possible. However, partial reconstructions—piecing together only certain aspects of what might have taken place—can be extremely valuable in putting together a more complete picture at a later time. Information developed through partial reconstruction at the earliest time possible, with a more complete process at a later date, often leads to a successful conclusion regarding whether or not a police officer was justified in opening fire.

It cannot be overly stressed that investigators and laboratory personnel (as well as medical examiner personnel in cases of death) must cooperate fully to (a) document every important aspect of a scene, (b) carry out an analysis of the physical evidence seen and recovered, (c) conduct a thorough and unbiased investigation of the case, and (d) share all pertinent information for reconstruction. In other words, a team approach should always apply to each and every crime scene reconstruction, whether or not the shooting involves a police officer.

All the details covered in the sidebar apply to the case at hand. Moreover, the question of perceived racism particularly deserves our attention. The case of the shooting of Salmon might serve as an object lesson in how, through a fair and thorough investigation, to keep public outrage under control. By handling such a situation expeditiously in a sensitive, unbiased manner, a potential race riot can be defused. This is not to imply that police shootings (or beatings), in and of themselves, are ever to be taken lightly.

THE RODNEY KING CASE

In 1991 Rodney King, a black motorist, was severely beaten, tackled, and Tasered by four Los Angeles Police Department officers. Most of the incident was captured on videotape by a private citizen from his nearby apartment and was quickly dramatized on television. The beating became a rallying point in Los Angeles and even an international cause célèbre.

The officers (three Caucasians and one Hispanic) claimed that King appeared to be under the influence of PCP, a "dissociative" drug formerly used as an anesthetic agent that exhibits hallucinogenic effects. King, who was on parole from prison on a robbery conviction and had past convictions for assault and battery, had led police on a high-speed pursuit through several red lights and boulevard stops before being captured and wrestled to the ground.

The Los Angeles district attorney subsequently charged the police officers with the use of excessive force in the arrest. A year later—on April 29, 1992—three of the officers were acquitted by a jury of ten Caucasians, one Latino, and an Asian. The jury could not agree on a verdict for one of the counts on the fourth officer. The verdict was based in part on the first two seconds of a thirteen-second segment of the video that had been edited out by television news stations. The total length of the rather blurry video was one minute and thirty-one seconds. In those initial two seconds, King allegedly got up off the ground and charged one of the officers before being subdued. A continuous beating followed. At the trial, the officers testified that they tried to physically restrain a violent King prior to the starting point of the video but he was able to throw them off. In spite of the acquittal, many people argued that King's action did not justify his brutal beating. The general public was largely unaware of the testimony and the edited video footage.

The jury's decision was generally considered to be the spark that ignited the so-called Los Angeles Riots of 1992, popularly known as the Rodney King Uprising. Thousands of people, mainly young black and Latino males, rioted in the Los Angeles area over the six days following the verdict. Television coverage was near continuous, including a great deal of footage from helicopter news crews. Viewers across the world were shocked as parts of the city went up in flames. Open gun battles and rampant looting sprang up everywhere. A white truck driver, Reginald Oliver Denny, was dragged from his vehicle and severely beaten by an angry mob.

Fifty-three people lost their lives, many of them murdered, and approximately two thousand people were injured. About thirty-six hundred fires were set, destroying eleven hundred buildings. More than ten thousand people were arrested. Estimates of the material damage done varied from $800 million to $1 billion. In addition to the Los Angeles Police Department, ten thousand soldiers from the California National Guard and thousands from the United States Army and Marines were deployed to suppress the crowds. And concomitant riots broke out in other US cities, including Las Vegas, Oakland, New York, Chicago, Seattle, and Phoenix.

In retrospect many believed that the Rodney King verdict was the trigger, but other factors contributed to the unrest in Los Angeles: high unemployment in the area, which had been hard hit by a nationwide recession; a perception that the LAPD engaged in widespread racial profiling; and specific anger over the light sentence given to a Korean shop owner for the shooting of a young black woman.

Thus, it was not without a vivid precedent that Hartford authorities were uneasy about the Aquan Salmon shooting. The highly publicized Rodney King case and its aftermath; the Connecticut cases in 1969, 1997 and 1999; and other incidents seemed fresh in their minds. There was no question they had to act fast to neutralize seething reactions by the minority community and thereby defuse the potential for full-scale violence.

A fraternal organization of minority Hartford police officers—the Hartford Guardians—vowed to oversee the investigation. This organization, which had served as a liaison between the department and the minority community for thirty-two years, announced that the police chief had assured them access to the investigators' findings.

"It says to the community ... that we are here to safeguard their concerns," said its president.

And I, as both a forensic scientist and the state's commissioner of public safety, tried to help galvanize appropriate courses of action. I made my public statement, based on unassailable facts that Salmon had *not* been shot in the back, right away in an attempt to assuage those in the minority communities who were crying foul. Also, on the day of the shooting, my staff at the Forensic Science Laboratory and I were asked by the Hartford Police Department and the Chief State's Attorney's Office to study the case and submit a reconstruction report. (I will paraphrase this twenty-page document later in this chapter.)

In the meantime, Roger Vann, president of the National Association for the Advancement of Colored People, called for action against Officer Allan, who had been on paid administrative leave since the incident.

"We believe there is obviously a lot more to the story than is being revealed," Vann said. "We don't want to rush to judgment, but we believe some corrective action should be brought."[9]

INVESTIGATION REPORTS

Among many subsequent interviews, statements, and written reports, the key ones were those of (1) Officer Allan, (2) the victim's friend Ellis Thomas, and (3) the Hartford Police Department Evidentiary Services Division. The following is the official documentation, edited so as to minimize duplication and provide clarity:

REPORT OF OFFICER ALLAN

On Tuesday morning, April 13, 1999, Officer Robert C. Allan (08–16–71) completed a written statement/report involving his actions the morning of the 13th. Officer Allan stated he had been a sworn member of the Hartford Police Department since May 2, 1996. [He] stated he was working the north end on patrol … when at approx. 0200 hours he heard over his police radio, from a nearby officer, a report that a female citizen was robbed at gunpoint. The description was of 3 to 4 black males and at least two firearms. The complainant also described the suspects' vehicle as a two-door white Cadillac with Connecticut registration 397KRZ. Officer Allan stated he started monitoring traffic looking for the vehicle when other nearby units reported that several more citizens alleged being robbed at gunpoint by the same 3 or 4 black males and the same white Cadillac...at approx. 0210 hours while he neared Capen Street, he observed a white Cadillac traveling southbound approx. 100 yards ahead of him. [He] said he closed the distance and verified the registration and he advised dispatch of the registration, direction and vehicle description. [He] also observed 4 black males in the vehicle.... [At] the intersection of Enfield & Greenfield Street he observed the rear passenger, right behind the operator, turn and look at him.... [The] Cadillac then increased its speed to 35–45 mph south on Enfield Street...then turned sharply, without warning, into the driveway to 25 Enfield.... [He] advised dispatch of the vehicle's direction and...then activated his emergency lights and siren in an attempt to stop the vehicle. [He] also stated he was aware that this area of Enfield Street was a high-crime area with reports in the past of shots fired, drug trafficking and stolen vehicles being stripped and abandoned.

Officer Allan reported there was no illumination in this area and the only lights were from the Cadillac and the [cruiser's] high beams. [He] stated that shortly after the Cadillac got to the dirt portion of the driveway/alleyway, the driver jumped from the moving vehicle with the other occupants remaining inside the car.... [He] placed his cruiser into park and turned off the strobe lights to provide a clearer view of the area. [He] reported that he observed a gun in the right hand of suspect #1 [Thomas] as he ran in the direction of the fence. Officer Allan reported that he yelled to suspect #1, "Police, stop or I'll shoot." [He] stated that he repeated to the suspect to "freeze" and announced "police." Officer Allan said he withdrew his department issued pistol and began to pursue the suspect with his flashlight.... [He] described the suspect as wearing baggy blue jeans, a blue pullover top with a light shirt underneath. The officer stated that while the suspect/operator was fleeing he heard a gunshot sound from the right and slightly from the rear of his location. [He] said he immediately radioed "shots fired"...he did not see the other occupants exit the Cadillac but his view...was somewhat obstructed by a tree that was in front and to the right of him...his attention was now [focused] in the direction from where the shot was heard and watching the suspect with the gun by the fence.... [He] illuminated the area with his flashlight while he held the pistol in his right hand trained on the suspect by the fence.... [He] assumed a crouched position and was quickly turning his head...to the area he heard the gunshot... again yelled to the suspect by the fence to "freeze" and identified himself as a police officer. The suspect refused to comply with [the] commands and continued to climb the fence.... Officer Allan...could still see the gun in the suspect's right hand...at the same time he heard a person running towards him from the area of the gunshot. The sound of the footsteps blended with the sounds of rustling leaves and branches.... [H]e kept his pistol pointed toward the suspect on the fence but turned the flashlight in the direction of the person running towards him. [He] said the person was wearing dark pants and a green jacket. Suspect #2 [Salmon] sprinted from behind a large tree and came around at such an angle that hid [his] suspect #2's right side. Officer Allan stated he was just south of a group of saplings and in front of a large tree. [He] stated that he pointed his flashlight toward #2 and yelled, "Police, freeze or I'll shoot." [He] described suspect #2 as being only ten feet away. Officer Allan stated that suspect #2 did not comply with his verbal commands and [suspect #2] continued to sprint toward the fence. Officer Allan said that suspect #2 now raised his right arm from his belt line across his body from right to left in an upward motion toward him. [He] stated that suspect #2 was turned sideways with his left side toward Officer Allan and was in a position south of and past his position. Officer Allan stated that based on his training and experience, the movement of suspect #2 was "consistent and indicative of a firearm being drawn and aimed in anticipation of firing."

Officer Allan stated that "at this point, this officer feared that suspect #2 was going to shoot and kill this officer." [He] stated that while "seeing suspect #2's hand being raised" and while moving north himself, he fired one shot towards suspect #2. Officer Allan stated that after the shot was fired "suspect #2 continued to advance a step or two to his right, retreated and ran toward the chain-link fence." [He] said that he pursued ... and grabbed the suspect's jacket near the neck, between the shoulders with his left hand. [He] said he forced suspect #2 to the ground, face down and put his knee on the back of [him] as he continued to watch suspect #1, who was now on the other side of the fence in a crouched position facing Officer Allan ... he and [the] suspect were approximately 6 feet from the chain-link fence.

Officer Allan explained from the time he heard the gunshot that came from his right, to the time he fired his weapon, approximately 2–3 seconds elapsed in time. [He] stated he gave verbal commands to suspect #1 to "freeze" because [he] could not see suspect #1's hands. Officer Allan said that suspect #1 ran south toward Mather Street at which point Officer Allan gave commands to place his hands out in front of him which he did. Officer Allan stated he wasn't aware that suspect #2 was shot until he noticed blood coming from his mouth while he patted him down for a weapon. Officer stated he immediately radioed for an ambulance. [He] also stated he saw a third suspect sprint from the area of the Cadillac west toward Magnolia Street and he yelled to Officer Rivera to apprehend him, which he did. As more officers arrived, Officer Musgrave started to administer first aid to the suspect that Officer Allan had shot. Officer Allan stated he didn't know the whereabouts of the fourth suspect. [He] said that Sgt. Jobes then seized his assigned weapon and gave him a replacement.

INTERVIEW OF ELLIS THOMAS

On Tuesday, April 13, 1999, from 1430 to 1630 hours, Ellis Thomas
(01–10–84) was interviewed at the Hartford Police Department.
...[He] was under arrest at Hartford P.D. for conspiracy to
commit robbery...conspiracy to commit assault II...and robbery...and assault 2nd.

Thomas stated that on Monday night he was hanging out with
Robert Davis, Aquan Salmon and Dennis Faniel. Thomas said
around 10 PM a white lady in a two-door white Caddy pulled
up to them. In the car, Thomas said, was a guy named "Earl"
who [was] from the neighborhood. Thomas said he had seen
this white lady before, two times, because she rented out her car
to people for drugs...the lady asked Robert for drugs, but he
didn't have any, so Robert gave her $15.00. Thomas said that the
lady gave him the keys and she and Earl walked away to another
car that belonged to Earl. Thomas said the four of them (Davis,
Salmon, Faniel) all got into the car and he (Thomas) was
driving. Thomas said that they had three "lighter" guns with
them. The "lighter" guns [were] really cigarette lighters but
they looked like real .25 caliber guns. Thomas said the guns
were silver or chrome in color and they got the guns around 5
PM on Monday at the Puerto Rican Store at the corner of
Garden & Mather Street for $7.50 each. Thomas said that
Dennis, Aquan and himself had the guns. [He] said that they
were driving around when they saw a black lady wearing a
"jiggy" coat near Mather & Magnolia Street. This lady had
thrown bottles at them in the past so they were going to get her.
Thomas said that Robert was driving the Cadillac and they
pulled up next to her. Thomas said they all got out of the car
and Aquan came up behind the lady and hit her in the back of
the head with the lighter gun. Thomas said the lady started
swinging around a bag that she was carrying and she said she
was going to call the cops, so [he] said they all left. Thomas said

Robert was driving when the cop came up behind them on Enfield Street. Thomas said that Robert pulled into a driveway on Enfield Street and everyone was supposed to jump out. Thomas said he was sitting behind Robert, and Dennis was in the front passenger seat and Aquan was sitting behind Dennis. Thomas said the police car had its lights on when they pulled into the driveway and Robert left the car running. Thomas said that he jumped out of the driver's side door as well as Aquan and Dennis jumped out of the passenger's side. Thomas said that Robert said he wasn't getting out of the car. Thomas said he ran to the fence and hopped the fence and Aquan was right behind him. Thomas said he didn't know what happened to the lighter guns because he didn't have them. Thomas said that the cop had his gun out and he yelled to Aquan to stop but Aquan turned around real fast towards the cop and the cop must have thought Aquan had a gun too and shot him. Thomas said he hid in the bushes on the other side of the fence because he was afraid. [He] said he saw the cop bending over Aquan telling him that he was going to be all right and that he was trying to help him. Thomas said that about two minutes later the ambulance came. [He] said he hid in the bushes for about an hour until the dog found him.

REPORT OF THE HARTFORD POLICE DEPARTMENT EVIDENTIARY SERVICES DIVISION

On April 13, 1999, members of the...Evidentiary Services Division responded to the 25 Enfield Street scene. The scene was documented...with video, photography, and sketches. The scene was also canvassed by members of the Major Crimes Unit as well as members of the patrol division.

The suspects' 1984 Cadillac Fleetwood, white, two-door with CT registration 397KRZ, was found stopped against a small pile of asphalt with the headlights on, both doors open and facing in a westerly direction. A Hartford Police Department patrol vehicle (Unit 21) was found parked approx. 100 feet west of Enfield Street and approx. 25–30 feet east of the white Cadillac. From the driver's side door approx. 15 feet south was the clothing of the deceased. A Federal .45 caliber spent casing was found south of the Hartford Police cruiser. A bronze color butane cigarette lighter pistol was found on the front seat of the Cadillac. A second bronze color butane cigarette lighter pistol was found on the ground behind a tree on the south side of the chain-link fence on the property of 224–226 Mather Street, where Ellis Thomas was arrested.

The service weapon of Officer Robert Allan was secured at the scene by Sgt. Patrick Jobes of the Hartford Police Department. The weapon, a Smith & Wesson, model 4506-1, .45 caliber, semi-automatic, was found to have one round discharged. Officer Allan was found to have three fully loaded clips containing eight Federal .45 cal. Rounds and the weapon was found to contain eight live rounds, one in the chamber, seven in the clip.

The deceased (Aquan Salmon) who was at the hospital, and his accomplices (Robert Davis III, Ellis Thomas and Dennis Faniel) all had gunshot residue tests done while in custody at Hartford Police Department. The clothing of the four individuals was also seized as evidence.

On April 13, 1999, at 2:27 AM, the body of [a] young black male was transported to St. Francis Hospital. The unidentified male was pronounced deceased by Dr. Christy at approximately 2:56 AM. The deceased male was wearing a black ankle-monitoring bracelet with the numbers "4685980695."[10]

AUTOPSY REPORT ESSENTIALS

On April 13, 1999, an autopsy was performed on Aquan Salmon by
Associate Medical Examiner Malka B. Shah of the Office of
the Chief Medical Examiner in Farmington, Connecticut. Key
elements of the procedure as described in the Investigation
Report are as follows:

The autopsy revealed that the deceased died from a single gunshot
wound that entered the left lateral aspect of the back of the
chest [see pages 175–76 for explanation]. The wound was
located [16½ inches] vertically below the top of the head and
3½ inches horizontally left from the back of the midline. The
central perforation measures 5/8 inches in diameter.

The bullet track reveals entry to the left part of the back of the
chest passing through the skin and soft tissue. The bullet
passes through the seventh intercostal [between ribs] space
grazing the superior [upper] aspect of the eighth rib then
entering the left thoracic [chest] cage, passing through the
upper part of the left lower lobe of the lung, exiting on the
medial [inner] aspect of the left lower lobe of the lung. The
bullet enters the pericardium [membranous sac enclosing the
heart], enters the left atrium [upper chamber of the heart on
the left] just below the inferior pulmonary [lower lung] vein
on the left side, passing through the left atrium, through the
interatrial septum [membranous wall separating the upper
two chambers of the heart], and exits the lateral aspect of the
right atrium [upper chamber of the heart on the right]
slightly anterior to the auricular appendage [in front of a
small pouch shaped like a dog's ear], passes through the pericardium anteriorly [the front of the sac enveloping the heart],
enters the middle lobe of the right lung from its medial
aspect, and exits from its anterior aspect, passes through the
fourth rib on the right anterior aspect of the chest and exits
from the right lateral aspect of the anterior chest exit wound.

The bullet direction is from back to front, left to right, and slightly
upwards.

The bullet penetrated the left lower lobe of the lung, bilateral atria
and interatrial septum, right middle lobe of the lung.

The cause of death is Gunshot Wound of the Chest and the
manner of death is Homicide.[11]

RECONSTRUCTION REPORT

Finally, there was one remaining official document that I hoped would
shed additional light on the case: my sixteen-page reconstruction
report. It was formulated at the request of the Hartford Police Department and the Chief State's Attorney's Office. The date of the request
was April 13, 1999, and the date of the report was May 21, 1999. It too
is presented in edited and paraphrased form. (As in the previous
chapter, photographs are referenced but not included.)

The following materials were submitted for laboratory analysis and
review:

Crime scene photographs
Crime scene reports, 7 diagrams
Autopsy report of Aquan Salmon
Autopsy photographs
Smith & Wesson, .45 caliber pistol. Model 4506-1
One spent casing
One bullet-like projectile
Clothing of "Aquan Salmon"
GSR kits
Piece of brick
Weapon-like objects
Latent fingerprint lifts

After detailed study of the submitted evidence, incident scene photographs, and autopsy records, information related to the shooting incident can be categorized as follows.

REVIEW OF SHOOTING SCENE PHOTOGRAPHS

Photograph #1 depicts an overall view of the scene as it appeared on April 13, 1999.

Photograph #2 is a closer view of the shooting scene. A Hartford Police cruiser, CT registration 596HPD, was in view. A white-colored Cadillac was located in front of this police vehicle, as can be seen in this photograph.

Photograph #3 is an overall view showing the rear of the white Cadillac. Both doors of the vehicle are open. The Cadillac's registration plate "397KRZ" can be seen in this photograph.

Photograph #4 is a closer view of the passenger side of the Cadillac. Various items can be seen on the floor, including a paper bag, a cup, a piece of vehicle interior, and other objects. Keys can be seen in the ignition.

A close-up view of the front passenger seat is shown in photograph #5. A handgun-like object can be seen on the seat. A closer view of this handgun-like object is shown in photograph #6. The handle grip is reddish-colored and has a gold-colored skull design on the surface and a shiny metallic finish on the barrel. Other objects can also be seen on the car seat as shown in this photograph.

Photograph #7 depicts an overall view of a pile of clothing-like material which was located in the general area of the decedent. A white-colored sheet which was used to cover the decedent is also visible in this photograph. Blood-like stains were observed on this sheet and on various objects of clothing, as shown in photograph #8.

A large bloodstain pattern was noted on the ground adjacent to this area, as shown in photograph #9. Photograph #10 is a close-up view of this bloodstain area. These stains consist of a large pool of blood and smaller stains adjacent to the larger blood deposit. These stains are consistent with a direct contact, deposit-type bloodstain pattern.

Photograph #11 depicts the area where a spent shell casing was located at the scene. A close-up view of the casing is shown in photograph #12. This casing was subsequently submitted to the laboratory for analysis.

A second handgun-like object was located near the fence, as shown in photograph #13. This area is on the side of the chain-link fence opposite the Cadillac and the side where the shooting occurred. The close-up view of this handgun-like object is depicted in photograph #14. This object has a dark-colored finish.

An overall view of the front of the Cadillac is shown in Photograph #15. A pile of asphalt-like material is in front of the vehicle. The Cadillac appears to have been stuck on this pile of material. A close-up view of the front bumper region and its area of impact with the pile is shown in photograph #16. The height of this pile appears to be at least level with the bottom of the car bumper.

Photograph #17 shows the shooting scene as viewed in a northerly direction. A chain-link fence is across the grassy area, separating the vacant lot. On the opposite side, the Cadillac is visible to the left in the photograph. A large number of objects and various types of debris can be seen on the ground in the vacant lot. Photograph #18 is a view of the shooting scene taken in a southerly direction. A garage-type building is on the right. Pieces of concrete, rock-like objects and other debris can be seen on the ground in this area.

REVIEW OF AUTOPSY REPORT AND PHOTOGRAPHS

A review of the autopsy report of Aquan Salmon, prepared by Dr. Malka Shah of the Office of the Chief Medical Examiner, and of the autopsy photographs that revealed the following information:

1. A wound was located in the back of the decedent, as shown in photograph #41. This wound was located approximately 1 foot 4.5 inches from the top of the head and 3.5 inches from the midline. The wound was slightly oval in shape, as seen in photograph #42. This wound was consistent with an entrance gunshot wound.
2. A wound was also located on the decedent's upper right chest just above the right nipple, as shown in photograph #43. This wound was approximately 1 foot 4 inches from the top of the head and 4 inches from the midline. A close-up view of the chest wound is shown in photograph #44. This injury was consistent with an exit gunshot wound.
3. The bullet track was determined to be from the left back through the body, exiting the upper right chest. The bullet trajectory within the decedent's body was from left to right, back to front, and slightly upwards.
4. An electronic monitoring device was identified on the right ankle of the decedent as shown in photograph #45. A view of this device after it was removed from his ankle is shown in photograph #46.

SCENE RECONSTRUCTION

On April 14, 1999, a briefing was given to Laboratory personnel at the Hartford Police Department by Chief Joseph Croughwell. Subsequently, Laboratory personnel were taken to the shooting scene. Present were Commissioner Dr. Henry Lee; Assistant Director Kenneth B. Zercie; Supervising Criminalist Robert O'Brien; Criminalists Thomas O'Brien, Edward Jachimowicz, Nicholas Yang, Jennifer Hintz; and Forensic Photographer Mark Newth. Also present at the scene were Hartford Police personnel, representatives from the Hartford and Chief State's Attorneys Offices, Dr. Shah and personnel from the Office of the Chief Medical Examiner, members of the decedent's family, and community leaders of the Hartford community. The scene was reconstructed with the assistance of the Hartford Police Department Major Crime Scene Unit.

The approximate position of the white Cadillac was determined and marked off with strings, based on the scene diagram and original Hartford Police Department photographs. Photograph #47 depicts this area as marked.

The approximate location of the .45 caliber spent cartridge casing, which was depicted in photograph #12, was also determined based on the original scene information.

Based on the results of the ejection pattern testing, the most likely position of the shooter was reconstructed. This was marked with a yellow marker "1" as shown in photograph #48. Photograph #49 depicts the location of this marker relative to the general scene location.

Based on the reconstructed position of the shooter, the possible field of view of the officer was determined. Some physical obstructions present at the scene limited the possible scope of the officer's view and movement of the decedent. A tree was located in a northerly direction, to the officer's right, as shown in photograph #50; a garage and fence were to the left of the officer's immediate location, as depicted in photograph #51. Thus, the most likely area in which the incident occurred was within a 45 degree arc, as shown in photograph #52.

With the assistance of Dr. Shah, a mannequin was placed with probes to reconstruct the bullet track through the decedent's body, as shown in photograph #53. This mannequin was repositioned in the areas where the decedent was most likely located at the time of the shooting. Photograph #54 depicts the rods in the established position of the bullet track.

Based on the final position of the decedent and a laser-assisted determination of the trajectory of the bullet through the body, a line search was conducted along the most likely trajectory path of the bullet after it exited the decedent's body. Subsequently, Det. E. Soto of the Hartford Police Department recovered a lead projectile at the rear of the building located at 160–162 Magnolia Street. The overall view of the area where the projectile was found is shown in photograph #55. This projectile was located behind the front driver's side tire of a gray Chevette parked in this location, as depicted in photograph #56. A close-up view of this projectile is shown in photograph #57.

Based on the location of the projectile and reconstructed position of the officer, the most likely trajectory of the projectile was determined by string projection. A pink string was used to mark this trajectory through the mannequin and toward the back of the building, as shown in photograph #58. The direction of travel of the projectile was determined to be from east to west, at a slight upward angle of approximately 10 degrees. *The decedent was most likely shot when he was facing sideways, in a southerly direction.* [Emphasis added.]

Officer Allan was subsequently brought to the scene to describe his recollection of his position at the time of the shooting and to observe the results of the reconstruction. (See photograph #59.)

Conclusions

1. The shooting scene was in a vacant lot located at 25 Enfield Street, Hartford. This scene is consistent with a primary, outdoor shooting scene.

2. Upon review of the shooting scene photographs taken on April 13, 1999, and comparison of these to the condition of the scene as observed on April 14, 1999, it was determined that there were some changes to the scene during this interval. Several items of debris and vegetation were removed. A rock-outlined shrine with candles was also erected. However, those changes did not substantially affect the overall condition of the scene for reconstruction purposes.

3. It appears that in the early hours of April 13, 1999, Officer Allan of the Hartford Police Department was driving his cruiser and followed the white Cadillac (CT reg. 397KRZ) from Enfield Street into the vacant lot. The Cadillac was stopped due to an impact with a pile of asphalt and rock-like material.

4. Both the driver's side and passenger's side doors were open and the Cadillac['s] lights appear to have been on when the original scene photographs were taken. This information is consistent with the occupants having left the vehicle in haste.

5. The handgun-like object located on the front passenger seat of the vehicle and the handgun-like object located near the fence at the scene (submission #014 & #015) were examined by the Firearms Section and found to be non-functioning. These items were found to be butane cigarette lighters with pistol-look designs.

6. Aquan Salmon died of a single gunshot wound. Based on the medical examiner's report, the bullet track was from left to right, back to front, and slightly upwards.

7. A spent cartridge case was recovered by the Hartford Police Department. Firearms Section examination results identified this casing as having been fired from Officer Allan's service weapon, a S & W .45 caliber pistol (submission #002).

8. A lead projectile (#12) was recovered at the scene using the reconstructed trajectory determined on April 14, 1999. This lead projectile is consistent with the type of ammunition and caliber of ammunition used by the Hartford Police Department and submitted with the officer's weapon.

9. Trace fiber evidence was recovered from the lead projectile. Laboratory microscopic and instrumental analysis results indicate that these fibers and fabric are consistent with the fabric composing the upper clothing layers of the decedent.

10. Based on the Firearms Section examination, the fiber analysis results, and the blood testing results, it was determined that this projectile is part of the lead core of the bullet fired from Officer Allan's weapon.

11. Based on the examination of the scene photographs and the results of the ejection pattern experiment conducted using submission #002, it was determined the officer's weapon ejected casings to the right rear and at an average distance of twelve feet.

12. Based on the reported location of the casing at the scene and the ejection pattern test results, the officer's most likely position at the time of the shooting was determined. There was a slight discrepancy between the estimated location determined by the reconstruction and the officer's recollection of his location at the time of the shooting. However, both of these locations are in the same general area.

13. Examination of the clothing of Aquan Salmon failed to reveal the presence of gunpowder residue. This result indicates that the decedent was greater than forty-eight (48) inches from the muzzle of the officer's weapon at the time of the shooting.

14. Based on a description of the position of the Cadillac, the physical obstructions at the scene, the lack of gunpowder on the decedent's clothing, and the final location of the decedent, it was determined that Aquan Salmon was in an area between approximately 26 feet to the northwest and 12 feet southwest of the officer. Based on the locations of the recovered bullet and spent casing, the trajectory of the bullet was determined to be slightly upward at an approximate ten (10) degree angle, and in a westerly direction.

15. Based on the reconstructed trajectory, the location of the entry

and exit wounds, and the lack of gunpowder on the decedent's clothing, the most likely position of Aquan Salmon at the time of the shooting was in an area approximately 10 feet in front of Officer Allan. The decedent was in an upright position, facing in a southerly direction. He was shot from the left back and sideways. Relative to Aquan Salmon's location, the general direction of the shot fired by Officer Allan was from left to right and from back to front at an acute angle.

16. The scene reconstruction results indicate a slight discrepancy between Officer Allan's recollection of the incident and the determined location of where the shot was fired. However, the decedent's position and the reconstructed trajectory are consistent with the *general* locations as described by Officer Allan.[12]

So what happened that night? At about 2:00 a.m., a police officer on patrol in Hartford's north end received a report on his cruiser's radio. A female citizen had been robbed and pistol-whipped by four black males. The suspects fled the scene in a white Cadillac. Other nearby police units soon reported that several more citizens had been robbed at gunpoint, apparently by the same men. They drove away in a similar vehicle. Within ten minutes, the officer spotted the car with its four black occupants, and he gave chase, eventually following it into a driveway/alleyway in a high-crime area of the city. It was an area with a reputation for frequent gunfire, drug trafficking, and stolen vehicles being stripped and abandoned.

According to Officer Allan, the Cadillac slowed when it came to a dark vacant lot. The driver leaped from the still-moving car, brandishing a gun in his right hand. Two other men soon scrambled out; one of them was Aquan Salmon. The driver sprinted toward a chain-link fence. Allan withdrew his pistol and, from a crouched position, shouted, "Police! Stop!" He repeated the words. At the same time, he heard a shot ring out from the right. There, a person—Aquan Salmon—emerged from behind a large tree and darted toward the fence. He never reached that fence, for Allan shot him upon seeing what appeared to be a threatening motion.

Soon after that night, the question arose: Was Salmon shot in the back? It quickly became a sticking point among those in opposite camps. One camp, advocating for the victim, held that if the bullet hole was located in Salmon's back side, then it must follow that he had to have been shot straight in the back. The other camp—those advocating a forensic evidence approach—disagreed, saying that the bullet hole was off to the left of the backside, near the scapula (shoulder blade), and that the bullet entered his body at an acute angle, exiting his front side on the *right*. This indicated that the victim was most likely turning to his left when he was hit. In the dark lot, illuminated only by the officer's flashlight, Allan's split-second assessment of the situation was that Salmon was indeed turning to his left and preparing to fire at him. Allan yelled, "Police! Freeze or I'll shoot!" Salmon ignored the warning and instead raised his right arm from his belt line and across his body from right to left. Allan believed this indicated a firearm was being drawn and about to be fired at him.

THE DECISION

State's attorney Kevin Kane's decision would not be made until ten months after the shooting. Throughout that period, law enforcement sources familiar with the case were dogged in reminding the public that the investigation was exhaustive and would be thorough and unbiased. But anger in the black and Hispanic communities continued to escalate, while many in leadership roles tried to defuse the tensions and prepare for the worst eventualities if Kane's ruling were to clear Allan of any wrongdoing.

Joseph Croughwell, chief of an embattled Hartford police force, developed heart problems soon after the shooting and was replaced by Acting Chief Deborah Barrows, an African American professional known for her calming influence. Considered one of the department's most effective communicators, she spent most of her career in community outreach and victim advocate roles.

"It was Deborah Barrows and company who kept the lid on the city when Aquan Salmon was killed," said Cornell Lewis, a substance abuse counselor and copastor of Hartford's North End Church of Christ. "She can take the pressure off whatever happens, and she'll have people in the community willing to back her."[13]

Croughwell offered his assessment of his replacement, stating that her mobilization of community leaders in the wake of the Salmon shooting, coupled with her visits to the Salmon family and talks with angry friends, helped the department and the city to weather the situation.

At the same time, the Center for Conflict Transformation was established in Hartford as a direct consequence of the shooting. The center was run by a multiethnic board of directors, all of whom were trained in conflict-mediation skills.

On February 15, 2000, the day before the release of the prosecutor's ruling, Sergeant Michael Wood, head of the city's 480-member police union, said, "You won't see storm troopers out there."

In my capacity as commissioner of public safety and state police, I issued a statement: "Some state troopers will be standing by, but we would only come in if Hartford police made a special request." I also indicated that the Salmon family would be notified before the ruling was made public. "Everybody is doing their best, I'm sure, to have the family and the community in mind," I said.[14]

The next day, February 16, was one that Kane and I will probably never forget. I left my home at 4:00 a.m., met with Kane and the chief state's attorney, Jack Bailey. We then briefed the governor about our findings. At 8:00 a.m., we met with Aquan Salmon's grandmother, the other members of his family, and the family's attorney to inform them of the major findings and the ruling. Although it was a ruling the family had not wanted, they appreciated our efforts, our sincerity, and our desire to meet with them before releasing the information to the media. Next we met with Hartford's community and religious leaders and pointed out the scientific facts behind the decision. The majority accepted our findings and conclusions, while a few brought up issues of bias and cover-up. However, we all agreed on the importance of overall community reaction in a case like this, realizing that the last thing anyone wanted was for riots to break out. Fortunately, none did, and I must thank many of the city's leaders for their efforts in this regard.

At 9:00 a.m., we addressed hundreds of Hartford's residents and media representatives who had assembled in a local church for a news conference. I can still recall the feeling of tension in the air when Kane, Barrows, and I walked past scores of TV trucks and cameras and into the meeting room. More TV cameras were inside, among a standing-room-only crowd. Kane first gave a few introductory remarks about the shooting and then played the police 911 tape of the communication between Allan and the operator. I followed with a discussion of the death scene investigation and the reconstruction of the shooting accident. I showed a PowerPoint presentation that included scene photographs and physical evidence and covered many of the scientific facts of the case. Kane ended the conference by spelling out investigative specifics in a narrative and appendix that totaled more than two hundred pages. Finally, he announced his ruling: Officer Allan had acted without wrongdoing.

POSTSCRIPT

In the final analysis—as we scientists are wont to say—this was a case that addressed the important issues of (a) the kind and extent of force required of police officers to apprehend lawbreakers; (b) the need for rapid assessment of the circumstances, particularly when disparate races are involved; and (c) the benefits of full cooperation between state and federal agencies in resolving potentially explosive situations.

The general consensus was that police representatives did a commendable job under trying circumstances. Most believed that community leaders did an excellent job of maintaining a cool temperature during the hot summer, despite constant criticism from some in the community. Moreover, many have said that scientists from the Connecticut State Forensic Science Laboratory and Connecticut State

Police Major Crime detectives played pivotal roles in scene reconstruction and reinvestigation of the shooting incident. It is my hope that despite lingering resentment in some quarters and demands for a federal inquiry in others, the handling of the case has served as a model for other law enforcement jurisdictions.

And what about the performance of Kevin Kane, who was appointed by the governor to rule on the case? It brings to mind *Mr. District Attorney*, a classic radio program of the 1940s. Each weekly episode began with a voice in an echo chamber: "And it shall be my duty as district attorney not only to prosecute within the limits of the law all persons accused of crime perpetrated within this county, but to defend with equal vigor the rights and privileges of all its citizens."[15] Kane fulfilled that duty.

In 2004 Governor M. Jodi Rell appointed Kane the chief state's attorney of Connecticut. As for me, I have retired from state service for the third time. But I was asked by the governor to stay on as chief emeritus of the Forensic Science Laboratory. My annual salary? One dollar.

ATROCITIES IN BOSNIA AND CROATIA

N
ext, we will investigate murders of a different kind—thousands of them. Let us begin with a history of the region involved, a history as convoluted as any ever recorded. We offer, however, an abridged version, remembering that the primary intent of this chapter is to describe my experiences in Bosnia and Croatia as they relate to the atrocities there. A secondary intent is to provide clarification to those readers who have heard of the breakup of Yugoslavia and its attendant atrocities but are not clear on precisely how they came about. Thus, to help navigate through the complexities, we begin with some background.

BACKGROUND

Yugoslavia, Then and Now

In the sixth century, groups of Slavs began to move into the Balkans—the southeastern European peninsula between the Adriatic and Black seas, stretching from Hungary to Greece. Calling themselves South Slavs, they migrated from what is now Russia and southern Poland. Each group soon formed its own independent state: the Serbs, Croats, and Slovaks established Serbia, Croatia, and Slovenia, respectively. But by 1400, foreign powers moved in and controlled nearly all of their land: The Ottoman Empire (based in present-day Turkey) ruled Serbia, Hungary occupied Croatia, and Austria took over Slovenia. The Ottomans also ruled Bosnia and Herzegovina at the time.

Four hundred years later, a movement for Slavic unity began. France's Napoleon Bonaparte brought about the unification of Croatia and Slovenia in 1809. However, six years later they were formally returned to the rule of Austria and Hungary. Serbia gained independence from the Ottoman Empire in 1878, but Croatia and Slovenia couldn't loosen the grip of Austria-Hungary, which, in addition, annexed Bosnia and Herzegovina. It had become a game of Who Rules Whom, and When?

During the early 1900s the movement to unite the South Slavs gained momentum. In 1914 a Serb assassinated Archduke Franz Ferdinand of Austria-Hungary in Sarajevo, the capital of Bosnia-Herzegovina. This led to a chain of events that ignited World War I, and when Austria-Hungary was defeated in 1918, the South Slavs were free to form their own state. Three political entities followed successively in the Balkans.

The name "Yugoslavia," which means "Land of the South Slavs," derives from the fact that in 1918, the first country to be known by this name was the Kingdom of Yugoslavia, which was created to unite Serbs, Croats, and Slovenes. It was invaded by the Axis powers in 1941 but was officially abolished in 1945.

The second country known by that name was actually renamed three times: Democratic Federal Yugoslavia in 1943, Federal People's Republic of Yugoslavia in 1946, and Socialist Federal Republic of Yugoslavia (SFRY) in 1963. In that year, its constituent republics were Slovenia, Croatia, Bosnia and Herzegovina, Montenegro, Macedonia, and Serbia (including the autonomous province that was eventually called Kosovo). But in 1991 the SFRY crumbled after a series of wars during which most of the republics declared their independence.

And the third country to bear the name was the Federal Republic of Yugoslavia (FRY) beginning in 1992. It consisted as a federation of the two remaining (i.e., nonsecessionist) republics: Serbia (including the autonomous Kosovo) and Montenegro. Once again, however, there was a name change, from FRY to State Union of Serbia and Montenegro. The name "Yugoslavia" was therefore officially abolished, and in 1996 the two constituents respectfully declared their independence, ending the last remnants of a Yugoslav state.

As we have seen, Yugoslavia's confusing mosaic of diverse peoples, languages, religions, and cultures evolved over centuries of conflict. But, as noted at the outset of this chapter, my main purpose here is to describe my role in the excavation and identification of hundreds of bodies in the eastern hillsides of Bosnia in the mid-1990s. These discoveries and relevant physical evidence would later be used to build a case against suspects indicted by the International War Crimes Tribunal in The Hague—suspects with names like Slobodan Milosevic, Ratko Mladic, and Radovan Karadzic.

But before I can relate my experiences, we still need to trace more history in the region. Let us examine the landscape around the time of World War I. At the war's end in 1918, the Central Powers of Germany, Bulgaria, Austria-Hungary, and the Ottoman Empire stood roundly defeated. Immediately, various South Slavic territories were cobbled together to produce a loosely knit Kingdom of Serbs, Croats, and Slovenes. Ten years later, King Alexander I renamed the country Yugoslavia and tried to curb separatist passions, but he was unsuccessful because of developments in Germany and Italy when Nazis and Fascists rose to power, and in the Soviet Union when Joseph Stalin became absolute ruler. Eventually the king was assassinated in Marseille by a Macedonian revolutionary.

Fast-forward now to World War II, when, in 1941, the Axis powers of Germany, Italy, Hungary, and Bulgaria attacked Yugoslavia, quickly occupied it, and split it up. More than three hundred thousand Yugoslav soldiers were taken prisoner. An Independent State of Croatia was established as a Nazi puppet state that soon created concentration camps for antifascists, communists, Serbs, Jews, and Gypsies.

Many resistance groups arose, such as the Chetniks, who became allies of the United States in Europe, and the communist Yugoslav National Liberation Army (NOV), led by Josip Tito, a Croatian

national. At first the army of Chetniks was highly successful in its guer-
rilla warfare, but then its efforts were dampened as German reprisals
against the Serb population became known: For every soldier killed, the
Germans executed one hundred civilians, and for each wounded, they
executed fifty. However, the NOV carried on fighting—but with staggering losses. Official Yugoslav authorities claimed 1.7 million casualties, most of them Serbs who lived in Bosnia and Croatia, as well as
Jewish and Gypsy minorities.

A series of hastily drawn conventions and resistance tactics by the
communists helped NOV expel the Axis from Serbia in 1944 and from
the rest of Yugoslavia in 1945—all of this in the face of intense occu-
pation efforts by the Germans. The Russians assisted in the liberation
of Belgrade but withdrew its troops after the war was over. And when
that time arrived, the new Federal People's Republic of Yugoslavia
was established, modeled after the Soviet Union, with Belgrade as its
capital.

As a reference, the complete names of the republics and provinces
mentioned previously are:

Socialist Republic of Bosnia and Herzegovina
Socialist Republic of Croatia
Socialist Republic of Macedonia
Socialist Republic of Montenegro
Socialist Republic of Serbia (which also contained the Socialist
    Autonomous Province of Kosovo and the Socialist Autonomous
    Province of Vojvodina)
Socialist Republic of Slovenia

Today each of the republics, with the exception of Bosnia, represents a distinct ethnic group, using its own language and maintaining its
own cultural identity. But it has not been easy. After Tito's death in
1980, ethnic tensions grew. There was an increase in nationalism
throughout the region: Slovenia and Croatia demanded looser ties
within the federation, Serbia sought absolute dominion over

Yugoslavia, the Albanian majority in Kosovo demanded the status of a republic, and many Serbian communities within Croatia rebelled and tried to secede from the Croat republic.

Slobodan Milosevic

Enter Slobodan Milosevic. Milosevic studied law at the University of Belgrade and became a successful businessman and banker. He bided his time in these occupations until, in 1984, he became head of the Communist Party in Belgrade and, three years later, led the Serbian Communist Party. It was a propitious time for him, as Serbian nationalism was on the rise following the fall of the Berlin Wall and Soviet communism. Challenging the Yugoslav federal government in a unique populist style, he won over thousands of supporters—especially with his socialist policy initiatives—and became an overnight hero in Serbia when he went to Kosovo to calm the fears of local Serbs amid a strike by Kosovar Albanian miners. In a famous speech televised throughout Serbia, he told the masses of angry people, "You will not be beaten again." In point of fact, very few Serbs had been beaten or even oppressed in Kosovo at the time, but this did not matter to 8 million Serbs who harbored deep historical grievances and welcomed a strong figure who might restore their place in history. Within a year—in 1998—Milosevic replaced party leaders in Kosovo and Vojvodina, and a year after that he became president of Serbia.

On the six hundredth anniversary of the Battle of Kosovo, in which the medieval Serb kingdom was defeated by Ottoman forces, Milosevic presided over a massive rally of more than a million Serbs at Kosovo Polje, the exact location of the historic battle fought in 1389. One of his first acts after this historic event was to rescind the autonomy enjoyed by Kosovo and to institute martial law in its place. Serbian nationalism was on the march. Kosovar Albanians were fired from their jobs, their schools were closed, they were denied access to state-run healthcare, and they lost administrative control of the province. This ushered in a decade of hell for the south Balkans. Milosevic and other Serb ultranationalists embarked on a campaign to create a Greater Serbia, unifying under one nation all areas where Serbs lived by driving out all minorities through a genocidal process euphemistically called "ethnic cleansing."[1]

As his reign wore on, Milosevic resisted political and economic reforms, multiparty elections, and moderate federalist policies. Clearly he wanted to abolish the confederation, and it did not take long for that to happen. Mounting tensions led to Croatian and Slovenian declarations of independence in 1991 and the secession of the Croats and the Muslims in Bosnia and Herzegovina in 1992. He backed Serbian rebels throughout the three-year civil war that ensued.

The last decade of Milosevic's life was marked by crisis and political upheaval:

> Suffering economic crises and the effects of sanctions, he signed a peace agreement in 1995, ending the civil war in Bosnia. He became president of the new Federal Republic of Yugoslavia, consisting of Serbia and Montenegro, in 1997. Ethnic violence and unrest continued in 1997 and 1998 in the predominately Albanian province of Kosovo, as a period of nonviolent civil disobedience against Serbian rule gave way to the rise of a guerrilla army.
>
> In March 1999, following mounting repression of ethnic Albanians and the breakdown of negotiations between separatists and the Serbs, NATO began bombing military targets throughout Yugoslavia, and thousands of ethnic Albanians were forcibly deported from Kosovo by Yugoslav troops. In June, Milosevic agreed to withdraw from Kosovo, and NATO peacekeepers entered the region. Demonstrations in the latter half of 1999 against Milosevic failed to force his resignation. Meanwhile, Montenegro sought increased autonomy within the federation and began making moves toward that goal.
>
> During the summer of 2000, Milosevic called for early elections, hoping to beef up his democratic façade. His plan backfired,

however, and voters elected the opposition candidate Vojislav Kostunica, a constitutional lawyer. Milosevic initially refused to concede defeat but resigned after several hundred thousand Serbs took to the streets in nonviolent protest to demand the end of his thirteen years of rule.

The already disgraced leader faced further humiliation in April 2001, when he was arrested after a twenty-six-hour armed standoff with police at his Belgrade home. He was charged with corruption and stealing state funds during his reign. Milosevic surrendered after Yugoslav officials promised him that he would have a fair trial and would not immediately be turned over to the United Nations War Crimes Tribunal at The Hague. He was, however, turned over to the UN in June. He was charged with committing crimes against humanity in Kosovo and Croatia. In November the UN War Crimes Tribunal charged him with genocide. *The indictment stemmed from his alleged activity during the 1992–1995 Bosnian war.* [Emphasis added.] He is the first head of state to face an international war crimes court. In his trial, which began in 2002, Milosevic defended himself. He died of a heart attack in March 2006 at the UN detention center at The Hague. His death precluded a verdict in his four-year trial, leaving open wounds and dashed hopes that he would be held accountable for the deaths of more than 200,000 people.[2]

The trial has been called the most important war crimes trial since Nazi leaders were prosecuted in Nuremberg, Germany, after World War II. And although Milosevic died before its conclusion, his legacy remains vast—and appalling. It is said that he brutalized people for at least a decade: A quarter of a million dead in Bosnia alone, and more than 3 million refugees. He "planned, instigated, ordered, committed or otherwise aided and abetted in a campaign of terror and violence directed at Kosovo Albanian civilians," according to the 1999 war crimes indictment against the former Yugoslav dictator. It was only part of the toll exacted during the leadership of the man known as "the Butcher of the Balkans."[3]

But aside from his unspeakable crimes, there is something more to be said about this man, and it was captured best on the first day of his trial by Chief Prosecutor Carla Del Ponte: "Beyond the nationalist pretext and the horror of ethnic cleansing, beyond the grandiloquent rhetoric and the hackneyed phrases—the search for power is what motivated Slobodan Milosevic."[4]

Extent of the War Crimes

Any consideration of the Bosnia/Croatia situation in the 1990s must include the parallel atrocities in Kosovo during the same time period. As that decade wound down, Del Ponte told the UN Security Council that her office had received reports that more than eleven thousand people were buried in five hundred killing sites in Kosovo, but that other categories of victims must be added to the list to get a sense of the scope of the human carnage. These include (1) those buried in mass graves in unknown locations, (2) a significant number of sites where the precise number of bodies could not be counted, and (3) victims whose bodies were burned or destroyed by Serbian forces. It was generally well known that such forces systematically erased evidence of massacres throughout Kosovo and even in Serbia proper, using means such as reburying bodies. Thus the number of bodies buried, burned, or otherwise destroyed may never be known, although a best estimate is that around ten thousand Kosavar Albanians were killed by Serbian forces.

A 1999 US State Department report titled *Ethnic Cleansing in Kosovo: An Accounting* identifies other human rights and humanitarian violations in Kosovo—that is, in addition to death itself.[5] The information was compiled from refugee accounts, documentation by nongovernmental organizations (NGOs) of the UN, press accounts, and declassified information from government and international sources. More than 1.5 million Kosavar Albanians—at least 90 percent of those living there at the time—were forcibly expelled from their homes. Moreover, tens of thousands of homes in twelve hundred cities, towns, and villages were damaged or destroyed. During the conflict, Serbian forces and paramilitaries implemented a highly organized "ethnic cleansing" campaign.

Multiple Definitions of "Ethnic Cleansing"

There is considerable controversy over the exact definition of the phrase "ethnic cleansing"—and even over when it all began. It really is a blanket term, and no specific crime goes by that name, but it covers a host of criminal offenses. One thing is certain: It is nothing new, as will be seen when we trace its origins below.

The most basic definition is that it is a process in which the advancing army of one ethnic group expels civilians of other ethnic groups from towns and villages that it conquers in order to create ethnically "pure" enclaves for members of its own ethnic group. Sometimes, in a bizarre but useful psychological twist, refugees of a group previously "cleansed" from their homes are forced to live in freshly "cleansed" territories of the conquering group. The vengeance and hatred felt by the displaced group sometimes manifests itself in ineffective acts of retaliation. These in turn serve the conquering leaders as a pretext for continuing what can only be termed "war crimes."

In the Bosnian war alone (1992–1995), ethnic cleansing created more than 2 million refugees and displaced persons. And this number increased with the expulsion of Serbs from Croatia and the savage atrocities committed by the Serbs against the Albanian majority in Kosovo prior to, during, and probably in spite of NATO air strikes. Although Serbs were by far the most successful "cleansers," all sides adopted this method in the course of the war.

It is fairly well documented that the same five steps were followed by all perpetrators, especially the Serbs:

- *Concentration.* Surround the area to be cleansed and, after warning the residents and urging them to leave or at least to mark their houses with white flags, intimidate the target population with artillery fire and arbitrary executions, and then bring them out into the streets.

- *Decapitation.* Execute political leaders and those capable of taking their places, including lawyers, judges, public officials, writers, and professors.
- *Separation.* Separate women, children, and old men from men of "fighting age"—sixteen to sixty years old.
- *Evacuation.* Transport women, children, and old men to the border, expelling them into a neighboring territory or country.
- *Liquidation.* Execute fighting-age men; dispose of bodies.

All of the largest atrocities of the Balkans war were variations on this gendercidal theme—targeting males capable of fighting.[6] These were the worst acts of mass killing in Europe since the killing of tens of thousands of disarmed enemy men by Tito's partisan forces in 1945 and 1946. A particularly monstrous incident occurred in Vukovar, a city in eastern Croatia, for example, when Serbs pulled hundreds of hospital workers and lightly wounded soldiers out of their hospital surroundings—some with catheters still dangling from their arms—executed them, and buried them en masse outside city limits.

But larger in scope was a more obscure event at Brcko, in Bosnia and Herzegovina, during the Serb offensive of 1992. Although much about the incident remains shadowy, the area appears to have been the target of systematic gender-selective slaughter that strongly foreshadowed the nightmare at Srebrenica three years later. In an article for the *New York Review of Books*, Mark Danner wrote:

During the late spring and early summer of 1992, some three thousand Muslims . . . were herded by Serb troops into an abandoned warehouse, tortured, and put to death. A U.S. intelligence satellite orbiting over the former Yugoslavia photographed part of the slaughter. "They have photos of trucks going into Brcko with bodies standing upright, and pictures of trucks coming out of Brcko carrying bodies lying horizontally, stacked like corkwood," an investigator working outside the U.S. government who has seen the photographs told us.... The photographs remain unpublished to this day.[7]

The crowning act of gendercide in the Balkans war took place in 1995, as reported by Adam Jones:

After the atrocities of 1992 and further fighting in 1993, Srebrenica had been declared one of the five "safe areas" under U.N. protection. [Many] thousands of desperate Muslims sought protection there. Despite privations and squalor, the safety held until July 1995, when Serb forces overran the enclave. As Dutch U.N. troops and the international community looked on, the Serbs separated the men... from the children and women. While the other members of the community were bused to safety in Muslim-held territory, [an estimated 8,000 Bosniak men and boys] were taken out to open fields, executed, and buried in mass graves. Thousands of other unarmed men were rounded up and hunted down in nearby forests, in what Serb commander Ratko Mladic called a "feast" of mass killing.

Jones continued:

One must not overlook the men and occasionally the women who slaughtered the defenseless victims and buried them in the mass graves, or killed them in their houses and streets. Again, although extreme nationalism was evident in Croatia, Bosnia-Herzegovina, and Kosovo, it is the ordinary citizens of Serbia who have overridingly supported their regime in its campaign to build "Greater Serbia" over the graves of Muslims, Croats, and Kosavars.[8]

In a more targeted definition of "ethnic cleansing," prize-winning journalist Roger Cohen wrote an article citing the United Nations Commission of Experts' definition of "ethnic cleansing" as "rendering an area ethnically homogeneous by using force or intimidation to remove persona of given groups from the area." In a sweeping 1993 report to the Security Council, the commission indicated that the practice was carried out in the former Yugoslavia by means of murder, torture, arbitrary arrest and detention, extrajudicial execution, rape and sexual assault, confinement of the civilian population, deliberate military attack or threats of attacks on civilians and civilian areas, and wanton destruction of property. The commission's final report in 1994 added these crimes: mass murder, mistreatment of civilian prisoners and prisoners of war, use of civilians as human shields, destruction of cultural property, robbery of personal property, and attacks on hospitals, medical personnel, and locations with the Red Cross/Red Crescent emblem. The report further stated that perpetrators of such crimes are subject to individual criminal responsibility, and military and political leaders who participated in making and implementing the policy "are also subject to charges of genocide and crimes against humanity, in addition to grave breaches of the Geneva Conventions and other violations of international humanitarian law."[9]

"Silent ethnic cleansing" is a term coined in the mid-1990s by certain observers of the Yugoslav conflicts. Overtly concerned about Western media portrayals of atrocities committed in the wars—which generally focused on those perpetrated by the Serbs—those atrocities committed *against* Serbs were labeled "silent," insofar as they did not receive adequate and accurate coverage.[10] Since then, the use of the term has been broadened by some groups to fit their own purposes, such as both sides in the Northern Ireland conflicts, and those who take exception to the expulsion of ethnic Germans from former German-occupied territories during and after World War II.

Finally, the most vivid picture of ethnic cleansing was rendered by Cohen, who expressed it this way:

Ethnic cleansing—the use of force or intimidation to remove certain ethnic or religious groups from an area—was the central fact of the wars of Yugoslavia's destruction. *The practice has a method: terror. It has a smell: the fetid misery of refugees. It has an appearance; the ruins of ravaged homes. Its purpose is to ensure—through killing, destruction, threat, and humiliation—that no return is possible.* [Emphasis added.][11]

PERSONAL EXPERIENCES IN BODY IDENTIFICATION

Between October 8 and 13, 1995, I was part of a group of American forensic experts who traveled to Croatia and Bosnia under the sponsorship of AmeriCares, an international humanitarian aid group based in Connecticut. My colleagues on the trip were forensic pathologist Dr. Michael Baden, codirector of the New York State Police Medicolegal Investigative Unit; forensic pathologist Dr. Barbara Wolf of the Albany (New York) County Coroner's Office; Dr. Moses Schanfield, a DNA expert from Denver, Colorado; and Dr. David Rowe, professor of pediatrics at the University of Connecticut School of Medicine.

Also there during that time were our counterparts from Croatia, all professors of pathology at the Split Medical Center in Split, Croatia: Drs. Simun Andelinovic, Marija Definis-Gojanovic, and Dragun Primorac. I first met Primorac shortly after he had received his medical degree from the University of Split and had begun studies toward a PhD in human genetics at the University of Connecticut School of Medicine. He subsequently interned at the State Police Forensic Laboratory and concurrently worked on a DNA typing of human tissues and bone project under my direction at the University of New Haven. I vividly recall the first day we met at my Meriden forensic laboratory. A tall, handsome, young man entered the lab; as he extended his hand, he introduced himself as Dragun Primorac from Croatia.

In my former work as a police detective, I had developed an ability to draw on my instincts and a sixth sense to gauge and personify strangers. As a scientist, I developed an ability to utilize logic and factual analysis to evaluate the trustworthiness of people. Over my long career, I have developed a reliable and effective system to understand personalities and human relationships. I do not require the use of tools such as the polygraph or various psychological tests to characterize an individual. Immediately upon meeting Dragun, I knew that this was an intelligent, diligent, energetic, and ambitious young man. In my mind, I knew that one day he would become a leader in his country. And sure enough, upon completion of his PhD dissertation, he returned to Croatia and shortly thereafter was appointed Minister of Science, Education, and Sports. Through the years, Dragun has served and represented his country with the utmost integrity and passion.

That first day, his appointment with me was scheduled for only thirty minutes. That brief thirty minutes, however, quickly became one hour; that one hour became two hours; and that two hours became four hours. We ended up chatting for more than six hours about random topics: from a DNA discussion to ethnic cleansing; from karate to life in Croatia; from science to the history of the Balkans; and finally, from mass genocide graves to my involvement with his investigation into war crimes. It was most enlightening.

It was he, along with Simun Andelinovic, who thus familiarized me with the Balkan atrocities and convinced me to participate with other Americans in mass grave investigations there.

I was well aware of the history behind the atrocities there, and I was mentally prepared for what we might encounter—to a point. What I hadn't counted on was how the experience would change my whole perspective: So moving were our discoveries and so heart-wrenching were the stories told by families who had lost their loved ones that I was not fully prepared for what I'd hear or see. One day their loved ones were there; the next day they were gone. I saw beautiful houses burned or full of bullet holes. The destruction was unbelievable; the human suffering was unfathomable. This devastation drove home the fact that fame, fortune, and material things mean nothing compared to life. Life can be short. Now I appreciate my work even more.

Our goal was to identify the dead and, through so doing, to heal the living. In many instances we interacted with families who, for two or three years or more, had been holding out the hope that their loved ones might still be alive. Some had been misled, being told that their relatives had been taken prisoner. But when the truth was uncovered, those families were allowed some kind of closure, sad as it was. Put another way, many of the dead were not, by and large, victims of battle. They were deliberately and brutally killed—not because of what they had done, but for who they were. After months beneath the ground, many of the bodies were decomposed beyond recognition; still, we would never forget that each of them was someone's son or daughter, brother or sister, and that their exhumation brought a certain peace of mind to the bereaved. And I believe I speak for my American and Croatian colleagues when I say that we too felt a small measure of personal satisfaction not only in unearthing bodies and not only when we could establish body identification, but also in working with Croatian scientists so that they could proceed with the process of DNA identification of skeletal remains after we left.

One of the most important aspects of the investigation of these types of murder is the positive identification of the victims.

Human Body Identification

As a society, we have traditionally placed considerable value on the positive identification of the dead and presenting the body remains to their family for internment. With an intact body, identification is relatively simple and can be achieved in the following ways:

1. Direct viewing and identification made by a relative, friend, or acquaintance.
2. Fingerprint identification using comparison of postmortem fingerprints with known print records or searching the AFIC database system.

3. Personal identification marks such as scars, tattoos, or birthmarks.
4. Artificial body part identification. Some of these are serialized and therefore readily identifiable. Even a pacemaker has a serial number that can be traced back to the owner. Contact lenses and artificial breast implants may be less traceable.
5. Medical records comparison. Hospital records of surgical procedures, as well as X-rays and other technologies, may be useful.
6. Identification of the victim's belongings, such as clothing, jewelry, identification cards, photographs, and the like. This is a less direct method of identification, and because of the possibility of a mix-up, many authorities do not rely on this method alone. For example, in the 9/11 World Trade Center tragedy in New York City, a body found in the rubble was identified as veteran firefighter Jose Guadalupe. This identification was made based on a flat gold chain around the body's neck and on a medical X-ray. However, subsequent DNA results showed that the body was actually that of another firefighter, Christopher Santori.

If there is destruction or fragmentation of a body due to fire or another traumatic event, the techniques described above are less reliable. In such instances, forensic scientists resort to the following approaches:

1. Examination of body or skeletal remains by a forensic anthropologist. Depending on what bones are recovered, such an expert can provide information about race, sex, age, stature, and other special features. These will not provide a

positive identification in and of themselves, but when combined, for example, with highly individualized medical interventions, a forensic anthropologist's findings can prove to be invaluable. The forensic anthropologist can also assist in a determination of the cause and manner of death and of other factors related to it.

2. Identification using dental records. Forensic odontologists can make positive identifications from an X-ray of a person's dentition provided that antemortem (before death) films are available. Use of dental records assumes, of course, that the remains contain jaws with teeth.

3. Genetic marker typing of tissues or bone. ABO typing of tissues and bone has been used for human identification for decades. In the case of a single body or if there is a limited number of possible identities—as in a plane crash involving four bodies or a grave with two bodies—ABO blood grouping and isoenzyme typing can provide information for positive identification. On the other hand, if there is a large number of casualties or a mass grave, genetic marker typing will only narrow the field or eliminate some individuals entirely.

4. DNA typing. This technique has been used extensively in recent years in both criminal investigations and human identification as applied to either man-made or natural disasters. Both nuclear and mitochondrial DNA (mt-DNA) can be extracted from tissue or bone specimens for human identification purposes. The mt-DNA approach yields results that are not in themselves definitive, but in conjunction with other techniques and in a universe of limited identities, it helps make identification possible. The

success of DNA identification relies on an accurate universe of possible identities, or with known
DNA samples from a family or a DNA database
that can be searched.

To reach the grave site areas, we flew from New York to Zagreb, Croatia; next we met our Croatian colleagues, drove into Bosnia with a military escort, and then boarded Russian-made military helicopters to get to the graves. Every village we could see was completely destroyed. *Every village!* In some, smoke was still rising. I must admit that we were all a bit apprehensive, not knowing what to expect. When we drove through the border, for example, we had no idea what might happen. Having a Green Beret–type Croatian special forces unit escorting us did help some—as did the constant comfort accorded us by Simun Andelinovic and Dragun Primorac. But still, there was a gnawing uncertainty, especially after we heard news of nearby mine explosions and sniper fire.

Our Russian-made helicopter was of 1950 vintage. It looked as though it was held together with rubber bands and duct tape. But despite its appearance, we anxiously climbed aboard. The pilot turned on the ignition. The engine rumbled. The helicopter bounced up and down, and it shook side to side. After thirty minutes of what seemed like a helicopter rodeo, the pilot was finally able to get the vehicle air-borne. Its passengers cheered over the successful liftoff. Simun, Dragun, a military commander, and I were plotting the map and reviewing reports of where potential grave sites could be located. Michael, Moses, David, and the rest of the crew were chatting with the soldiers about this unique experience.

We flew over territory controlled by the Serbs. Throughout the ride, I heard various gunshots and explosions. When I was twenty-one years old, just after I graduated from the Taiwanese Central Police College, I was drafted to serve in the Republic of China army as a second lieutenant. In 1959 my unit was stationed in Kim Mung, a small island off the coast of China. During that period, tension between China and Taiwan was at its peak. Every day, both sides would fire at each other. Since then, I remain familiar with the sounds of artillery, rockets, and machine guns.

The military commander confirmed my conclusions about the sounds. He ordered everyone to remain seated. The cabin was dead silent as each passenger listened intently for the sound of gunfire, which was competing with the noise made by the helicopter's rotor blades. Peeking though the windows, we could see the explosions triggered by rockets. Our silence grew into fear.

To ease the tension, I asked the commander, "Why don't you tell the pilot to fly higher?"

"This is the highest we can fly," he replied. He assured us that he had flown over the region several times and had never been hit. Hearing that was a relief. Of sorts.

Simun turned to me and asked, "Dr. Lee, are you scared?"

I said, "No, I am not. I've always believed that when my number is up, it is up. However, the only thing I don't want to happen is for my number not to be up, but to have someone whose number *is* up to sit next to me." Laughter broke the silence.

We landed in an area controlled by UN soldiers. A military caravan picked us up and escorted us through a country road to the grave sites.

Our operation was based in Kupres, a Bosnian city about twelve miles from the Croatian border that was occupied by the Serbs in 1992. We worked with and lent support to Simun and Dragun as well as the forensic team from Split Hospital in the town of Split, Croatia. In keeping with our overall mission, we not only assisted in the excavation of bodies at mass graves and assisted at autopsies, we also worked with forensic teams in meeting with families to help them identify bodies. When we could, we spent time with the scientists in their DNA laboratory, which had been set up a year before. They consulted with me and I offered whatever guidance I could in helping them deal with those cases that could not be identified using traditional anthropological means.

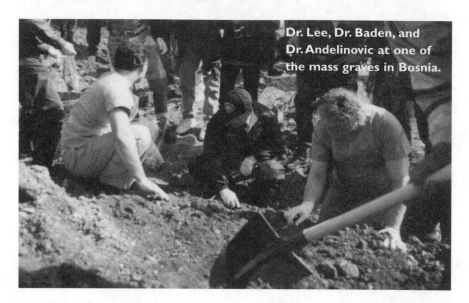

Dr. Lee, Dr. Baden, and Dr. Andelinovic at one of the mass graves in Bosnia.

At many of the grave sites we visited, the dirt had already been cleared from the bodies, but at some of them we dug down ourselves, finding three bodies in Petrinji, for example, and about fifty at a neighboring site—mostly elderly people, male and female. The most difficult part of the grisly task of exhumation was in separating the decomposed bodies into sets of bones, clothing, and other evidence that constituted single individuals. Additionally, the Serbs often buried land mines alongside victims or otherwise booby-trapped the graves. Luckily our timing was good, for we were told that before our arrival a dog had been blown up at a site by a land mine, and media reports noted that three antitank grenades were recovered at the site just hours before; presumably they had been placed there to prevent anyone from excavating the bodies. Obviously, the mines and grenades were of serious concern to us.

We learned that the bodies in that grave had been buried in 1991. They were found to be in bad shape because of both decomposition and an unsatisfactory burial process, so they consisted primarily of skeletonized remains or partial skeletons. And as we were examining these bodies, we were reminded by local authorities that there was ongoing violence nearby. In fact, an adjacent autopsy room was the site of autopsies of soldiers being killed in the current fighting. I should also point out that there was not always the "luxury" of an autopsy room per se; in many cases we had makeshift autopsy tables at the edge of a mass grave. Nor were the bodies extensively autopsied with great precision, simply because of the enormity of numbers. Although some traditional identification methods could be called upon in a few cases, the most common approach was direct viewing by families. In such cases we would arrange the bodies on tables in a way that we hoped would be the least grotesque to family members; for example, we might place a soldier's helmet over a large hole in his chest.

In total, it took us four days and four nights of steady work to identify thirty people—a small contribution compared to the bigger picture, but there wasn't much more we could do, at least with respect to the identification process itself. It was a tedious and saddening process.

I clearly remember the gratitude of the residents of Kupres, even when the news was bad: Vuatico Couc's daughter, Ivanica, was thirty-two when she died. She had been a teacher until she joined the Croatian Democratic Party and was fired by Serbian officials. Subsequently she became a journalist for Croatian newspapers, and the Serbs became even more incensed. Until I identified her remains, the family was uncertain of her whereabouts, whether she was a prisoner or dead. Her father said simply, "I just want to thank you, Dr. Lee... we wanted to know."

Contrary to what we had anticipated, only thirteen identifications were made through DNA genetic testing techniques, because most of the victims either had no blood samples on record to compare with, or their relatives (who could provide blood samples for DNA matching) had fled to far-flung refugee camps, or their bodies were simply too badly decomposed to extract any workable DNA. Instead, the Croatian scientists estimated the time of death and coordinated that with information gathered from family members, and with other anthropological methods such as estimating body size, height, and weight. So, in many instances, certain assumptions had to be made; I suppose you might call it extrapolating. Yet under the circumstances—that is, lacking valuable identification information such as dental or fingerprint records—it was all we had to work with. There were no birth or medical records; the hospitals were all gone. There were no antemortem records, so a lot of the usual identification techniques couldn't be utilized. There were no family photographs, no identifiable tattoos to examine. All we had to go on were things like body weight, height, jewelry, and clothing. Yes, clothing was *most* important. One victim's family said the man was wearing Nike socks. We found that man.

Local dentists helped out. They had no records anymore, but they often remembered doing a root canal procedure or pulling a tooth, so they would go through a victim's mouth. You can imagine how gruesome that was.

The groupings of the bodies in some of the graves cut across many lines: soldier and civilian, man and woman, adult and child. And while we were not looking for specific causes of death ("cause of death" refers to the disease or injury that produces a disruption in the normal functioning of the body resulting in the death of the individual; e.g., a gunshot wound to the head), it was apparent that most had died from multiple wounds, including gunshots and bayoneting. A special obstacle to a conclusive determination of cause of death was evidence that many of the bodies had been bulldozed and that attempts had been made to burn the bodies.

I must acknowledge that our counterparts in Croatia are pretty savvy—very advanced. And despite working under miserable circumstances, they held their heads high. They taught me quite a few things. I learned how to work in a mass grave under less than ideal conditions. I learned more about decomposition and its effects on the human body. These were things that would benefit me in my future work. The fact is that in my career I have seen more bodies at a single in time than here, for example, in an airline crash. But those bodies were fresher and therefore easier to identify. On the other hand, in the Balkans, some of the victims had been buried since 1991 and 1992.

That time period—that is, a few years before our visit—roughly coincided with the time when several of their scientists came quietly to my Police Forensic Science Laboratory in Connecticut to study for a month or more.

And several years after our visit—ten, to be exact—the *International Herald Tribune* reported that a team searching Bosnia's countryside for mass graves stated it had detected geological patterns that would help in locating graves in the future. The team, the International Commission on Missing Persons, presented the news at a mass grave site in Cancari, some sixty miles northeast of Sarajevo. The site was one of sixteen studied by experts in satellite imagery, geology, and forensic archeology for the Bosnia-based commission.

"We looked at a series of technologies that can be used in combination to help find mass graves," team leader John Hunter said. "We are not talking about some kind of magical grave detector, but about a system of techniques that will find patterns and differences in the ground that we know are associated with mass graves. This kind of work is all about finding those clues."[12]

The team's scientists, from the United States and Britain, found that such graves were characteristically located in river valleys, in the corners of meadows or fields, within 330 feet from a road, or on a slope from a road. Dense weeds and grasses usually overran the areas. Tests of soil resistance to electricity also revealed patterns that helped in finding the graves and in establishing their depths and composition.

Satellite imagery—photographs of planets (in this case, Earth) made by means of artificial satellites—and spectral analysis, which measures changes in ground surface composition, have also been used to find mass graves elsewhere, as in Iraq. Such technologies, which are noninvasive and therefore do not disturb the graves, also thwart any efforts to cover up evidence of mass killings.

"The combination of methods outlined in this study will help us find mass graves and will make it more difficult for perpetrators to hide mass graves in the future," said Jon Sterenberg, head of the Bosnian commission's Excavations and Examinations Division.[13]

But beyond the strictly scientific aspects of our mission, I discovered some other things, both in direct conversations with local officials and in subsequent communications with scientists we befriended there. In a sense, then, the voyage to the Balkans turned out to be a reciprocal affair, encompassing not only what they hopefully learned from us but also what we learned from them.

- We learned that at the time of our visit, there were at least 143 mass graves in Bosnia and 44 in Croatia, of which more than 100 were believed to contain victims of blatant genocide.

- We learned that human rights experts estimated that one hundred of the grave sites contained at least one hundred to five hundred bodies, and thirteen contained many more than five hundred. These are staggering numbers. The most infamous of the sites were those in the fertile valleys around Srebrenica, the so-called UN-protected safe area in eastern Bosnia that was overrun by the Bosnian Serb army. This locale of the worst known atrocity of the war commanded enormous international attention. However, it is one thing to be apprised of the situation while back in the States and quite another when you are physically in the area and are talking to those who lived it. Srebrenica galvanized international attention because of the enormity of the slaughter. (At the time of the slaughter, it is said, the international community did nothing and the UN peacekeepers looked on.) In addition, Srebrenica is remembered because General Ratko Mladic, commander of the Bosnian Serb army, and Radovan Karadzic, the Bosnian Serb political leader, were indicted for war crimes in connection with it and were made the subjects of international arrest warrants.

- We learned that local observers feared that the horrendous discoveries and attempts at identification as in Srebrenica would be repeated at other sites across the war-ravaged land. We were briefed that the slow and costly challenge to find all these sites may never be completed, for such are the practical and political realities of the situation. But the effort, including our own modest contribution, offered and would continue to offer new insights into the ways tens of thousands of civilians were killed during the war. Many of them were murdered in the towns and villages where they had lived peacefully alongside their Slav neighbors for years, even intermarrying, attending the same schools, and sharing festive occasions. It's beyond credulity how tears of joy and tranquility can suddenly be transformed into tears of unbearable grief.

- We learned that some officials held that it might be easier to forget the savagery than to proceed with further investigations that could only exacerbate tensions. The flip side of this, however, is that establishing the truth about what happened in the Balkans was essential not only for the sake of justice but also for the creation of a lasting peace. This was the view promulgated at the time by the UN, which argued that without justice the desire for revenge could trigger another full-blown war.
- We learned that according to human rights watchers, the exhumation of the mass graves was essential for recording humankind's potential and actual inhumanity. Not since Nuremberg, fifty years earlier, had there been such a systematic push to bring about prosecutions for war crimes.
- We learned that what happened following the fragmentation of Yugoslavia was not as far-reaching as Adolf Hitler's killing machine, but that the ethnic cleansing involved was not all that different. It was certainly smaller in scale, and in Yugoslavia, as opposed to the Holocaust, the drive was not to kill every man, woman, and child of a different religion. Clearly, though, the discovery of mass graves drives home the reality of the atrocities committed there.
- We learned that the vast majority of victims interred in the mass graves were Muslims killed by Serbs. However, as the UN investigators recognized, the Croats and Bosnian Muslims also carried out many atrocities.

As I look back on the experience, I can still picture the large-scale mass destruction of lives and property. At that time, in addition to the loss of life and limb, people had to live without the basic essentials, including electricity and water. And yet, despite their hardships and losses, they were gracious to us and tried their best to take care of us. I especially remember an occasion when villagers slaughtered a goat to make a large dinner for us. We drank so many bottles of wine, I lost count. It wasn't because we wanted to get drunk; rather, we merely wanted to keep warm in the middle of a winter without any heat. Somehow, I felt very bad about that. We volunteers on the US team tried, in turn, to be of help to them by giving their doctors and scientists support and positive reinforcement. Basically their techniques were good, but perhaps we made the group feel more comfortable. The most rewarding thing for them, I would imagine, is that the world did not forget them—the American people did not forget them.

GENOCIDE, GENDERCIDE, AND STORIES OF HUMAN INTEREST

The Balkan story does not stand alone as an example of humankind's potential savagery. Here are a few others taken from Gendercide Watch. (Gendercide, as discussed above, is the deliberate extermination of persons of a particular sex.) They have remained in the consciousness of many worldwide observers and cover a wide range of countries— from Iraq, Armenia, Bangladesh, India, and East Timor to Germany, China, Rwanda, and the former Soviet Union.

> The anti-Kurdish "Anfal" campaign, mounted in 1988 by the Iraqi regime of Saddam Hussein, was both genocidal and gendercidal in nature. "Battle-age" men were the primary targets of Anfal.... Throughout Iraqi Kurdistan, although women and children vanished in certain clearly defined areas, adult males who were captured disappeared en masse.... It was apparent that a principal purpose of Anfal was to exterminate all adult males of military service age captured in rural Iraqi Kurdistan. Only a handful survived the execution squads.

The Armenia genocide (1915–1917) was one of the most massive exterminations ever carried out against a defenseless people. In 1915, as World War I raged, the Turkish government (ruler of the Ottoman Empire) decided upon the systematic extermination of most of the male Armenian population, and the forced deportation of the remainder, mostly women, children, and the elderly. The deportation became a death march, with extreme violence and deprivation leading to the death of most of the survivors of the initial gendercide—as was intended. By the time the exhausted and traumatized survivors reached refuge in neighboring countries, up to three-quarters of the entire Ottoman Armenian population had been exterminated.

Genocide in Bangladesh (formerly East Pakistan) during nine months of 1971 stands out as one of the most concentrated mass killings of noncombatants in twentieth-century history. In an attempt to suppress Bengali independence forces, the West Pakistani military regime unleashed a horrific wave of slaughter that may have killed 3 million people. The mass rape and often the murder of Bengali women, along with children and the elderly, were accompanied by truly staggering atrocities against younger men, who constituted a large majority of the victims.

Case studies of the events in East Timor in September 1999 are arguably the most ambiguous of studies of gendercide. Indeed, it is impossible to state with certainty that a fully-fledged gendercide did occur, and on what scale. Nonetheless, in the opinion of many, there are grounds for believing not only that genocidal atrocities occurred during the period immediately following Timor's independence vote, but that they were widespread, preplanned, and systematic—and were also strongly gendercidal in character.[14]

The Holocaust inflicted upon European Jews by the Nazi regime was without doubt the most systematic and sadistic campaign of mass extermination ever mounted, resulting in the murder of 6 million Jews, as well as homosexuals and Gypsies. The Nazis killed and tortured women and men alike. They wanted to stamp out an entire "race," so they did everything they could to exterminate Jews of both sexes and all ages, unless they could be used for slave labor.

In 1937–1938 the Nanjing Massacre, also known as the "Rape of Nanking," represented another rare example of simultaneous gendercide against women and men. The massacre is generally remembered for the invading Japanese army's barbaric treatment of Chinese women. Many thousands of them were killed after being gang-raped, and tens of thousands of others were brutally wounded. Meanwhile, approximately a quarter of a million defenseless Chinese men were rounded up as prisoners of war and murdered en masse, used for bayonet practice or in experiments with toxic gases, or burned and buried alive by Japanese soldiers.

The 1994 genocide in the tiny central African country of Rwanda was one of the most intensive killing campaigns—possibly *the* most intensive—in human history. Few people realize, however, that the genocide included a marked gendercidal component; it was overwhelmingly selective, targeting Tutsi and moderate Hutu males. The gendercidal pattern was also evident in the reprisal killings carried out by Tutsi-led guerrillas during and after the mass slaughter.

In a mere eight months in 1941 and 1942, invading German armies killed an estimated 2.8 million Soviet prisoners of war through starvation, exposure, and summary execution. This little-known gendercide vies with the holocaust in Rwanda as the most concentrated mass killing of any kind in history—though not of the number of the Holocaust in Europe.

Under the dictatorship of Joseph Stalin, millions upon millions of ordinary individuals were executed or imprisoned in labor camps that were little more than death camps. Perceived political orientation was enough to get someone thrown into these prisons.

Dr. Lee's snapshots drive home the depth of some of human history's worst nightmares. But returning to the bloodbaths of the former Yugoslavia, there is no dearth of personal stories to learn from and remember. The following are at once depressing, insightful, and poignant. They are extracted from Stephen Talbot's *Srebrenica: The Video of a Wartime Atrocity.*[15]

(Anonymous)

> As a correspondent, I was witness to much of the aftermath of these events....Bosnia will never go away for those of us who saw it firsthand. It has been burned into our consciousness in a way that can never be exorcised....I think as the guilt of what happened continues its acid etch on the soul, we will...hear more of this. It is a caustic thing, something that must be lanced and allowed to drain.

Kip Reitz—Columbus, GA

> I served with the US Army patrolling Srebrenica in 1999, four years after the July 1995 atrocities took place....The thing I came away with mostly is a feeling that, on the verge of the 21st century, humankind had yet to learn a single thing about the need to live alongside one another peacefully and put petty differences aside. I know of no other creature in the natural world that seems as hell-bent on its own demise as the human race. And I don't think it will ever change.

(Anonymous)

> It is very sad that even when the Bosnians, Serbs and Croats left their homes to find safe harbour in accepting countries like

Australia, that when they arrived, they still could not learn to get along. In Australia, Serbians and Croatians cannot even play [in] sporting events without keeping the crowd separated so that they do not fight with each other.

(ANONYMOUS)

We must look to what precipitated these atrocities. Dig back to the past. What have we been taught as Muslims, Christians, Hindus, etc? It is dividing us all. Only MY GOD is right... everyone else is wrong!

(ANONYMOUS)

I have spent a lot of time in former Yugoslavia.... It is always the other person's shame and problem. Excuses abound. This is the true shame of the war.... [This] is a war of snipers, burning villages, rapes and attacks on plain-clothed citizens. This is not a proud war of heroes and patriots.

FINAL THOUGHTS

On a return visit to the region several months later, we met with the mayor and other dignitaries. He was eloquent in his praise for and appreciation of the efforts of all the forensic scientists who participated in the project.

I represented the US group by first thanking them all for their hospitality. Next I stressed my confidence that we scientists shared the following sentiments, which grew in large part from our visits there. I stated that the world is getting smaller day by day; that hours before we had been in the United States, and now we were once again in the midst of their battlefield. The words seemed to come easy for me because I felt so strongly about what I wanted to convey.

Unfortunately, due to religious, political, and regional differences, the massacres still continue. But why can't we learn from history? Why can't people everywhere live more peacefully—in harmony rather than in deadly discord? Although many people speak different languages, there is a common language called "Love and Caring." Why can't they find it, embrace it, and believe in it? If so—and if this common language could be shared—perhaps such widespread and unspeakable tragedies can come to an end.

EPILOGUE

This book differs from the others we have coauthored in at least two respects.

First, it contains the most diverse group of cases we have discussed to date. Chapters 1–4 feature an eclectic array of characters: a legendary but erratic music producer, the only Catholic priest ever convicted of murdering a nun in the United States, two teenagers whose twisted minds led them to mass murder, and a Caucasian police officer whose shooting of a young African American man nearly sparked a race riot. And the fifth and final chapter isn't about a case at all—it's about thousands of cases.

Second, we limited our previous books to crimes committed within the United States. In this one, however, we also ventured into Bosnia, Croatia, and the surrounding areas. We told of my experiences and those of my colleagues in helping excavate and identify body remains from mass graves. But beyond that, we tried to cast some light on a historical past that is as confusing and sordid as any ever recorded. In essence, then, our personal story enables us to convey the bigger picture, one too compelling to ignore. As authors, we have tried to trace historical events without sacrificing necessary detail and to portray the brutality and massive slaughter in the countries of eastern Europe for what it was—senseless genocide. For some who live in that region, what happened in Bosnia has been burned into their consciousness and will never go away. Others—those who try to understand why people cannot get along (in this case, Serbs, Muslims, and Croats)—remain generally baffled, but they seem to place blame on radical extremists who initiate and perpetuate hatred and ill will. They may be right. And among the lingering weariness and resentment, there are no doubt militaristic elements roaming the hills, plotting their next conquest. We shall see.

In the first four chapters, the disposition of the cases is varied. As of this writing, Juan Luna and Father Robinson are in prison; Phil Spector was found guilty in a retrial and was sentenced to nineteen years to life on May 29, 2009. Officer Allan has been cleared of any wrongdoing, and James Degorski was found guilty on seven counts of first-degree murder in September 2009.

On the brighter side, these cases highlight the value of both time-honored and new forensic technologies, whether they involve examination of gunshot residue, bloodstain pattern analysis, bullet trajectories, or DNA extracted from fourteen-year-old chicken bones. They also illustrate the tedious but steadfast work of police detectives.

We have seen how long it can take for justice to be done. But we have also seen how, using the tools of science, law enforcement makes every effort to ensure that such justice is eventually served.

NOTES

CHAPTER 1: THE PHIL SPECTOR CASE

1. "Phil Spector," Wikipedia, http://en.wikipedia.org/wiki/Phil_Spector.
2. Ibid.
3. "Wall of Sound," Wikipedia, http://en.wikipedia.org/wiki/Wall _of_Sound.
4. "Phil Spector," Wikipedia.
5. Ibid.
6. Associated Press, February 3, 2003.
7. Kurt Loder, "Phil Spector: Mad Genius," MTV News, February 4, 2003, http://www.mtv.com/news/articles/1459844/20030204/spector_phil.jhtml.
8. Ibid.
9. Associated Press, February 4, 2003.
10. *Los Angeles Times*, February 5, 2003.
11. Ibid.
12. Ibid.
13. Alhambra Police Department, Crime Report Narrative, February 3, 2003.
14. Autopsy Report, Los Angeles County Department of Coroner, February 4, 2003.
15. *Los Angeles Times*, February 4, 2003.
16. Ibid.
17. CourtTV.com, May 11, 2007.
18. FoxNews.com, February 4, 2003.
19. MTV Networks, March 12, 2003.
20. MTV Networks, June 4, 2003.
21. CourtTV.com, September 19, 2003.
22. CourtTV.com, November 15, 2004.
23. Ibid.
24. CourtTV.com, January 7, 2005.

25. CourtTV.com, May 24, 2005.

26. CourtTV.com, January 31, 2006.

27. CourtTV.com, October 28, 2005.

28. Ibid.

29. CourtTV.com, April 25, 2007.

30. CourtTV.com, April 26, 2007.

31. Ibid.

32. CourtTV.com April 25, 2007.

33. CourtTV.com, April 27, 2007.

34. CourtTV.com, May 25, 2007.

35. CourtTV.com, May 11, 2007.

36. CourtTV.com, May 16, 2007.

37. CourtTV.com, May 4, 2007.

38. Ibid.

39. CourtTV.com, May 17, 2007.

40. CourtTV.com, July 12, 2007.

41. ActressArchives, www.actressarchives.com, May 30, 2007.

42. CourtTVNews, August 29, 2007.

43. CourtTVNews, June 13, 2007.

44. CourtTVNews, June 22, 2007.

45. CourtTVNews, June 28, 2007.

46. Ibid.

47. Ibid.

48. CourtTVNews, July 26, 2007.

49. CourtTVNews, August 27, 2007.

50. CourtTVNews, August 31, 2007.

51. CourtTVNews, September 6, 2007.

52. letters@latimes.com, Dawna Kaufmann, April 1, 2009.

53. letters@latimes.com, September 7, 2007.

54. *Guardian*, September 27, 2007.

55. Ibid.

56. *Mail & Guardian On Line*, October 4, 2008.

57. Associated Press, March 24, 2009.

58. Ibid.

59. Associated Press, April 13, 2009.

60. Ibid.

61. *Los Angeles Times*, March 29, 2009.

62. Attorney Doron Weinberg and trial consultant Susan Matross, editorial response, *Los Angeles Times*, April 1, 2009.

CHAPTER 2: BROWN'S CHICKEN MASSACRE

1. Maurice Possley, *The Brown's Chicken Massacre* (New York: Berkley Books, 2003), pp. 24–28.

2. *Chicago Tribune*, March 27, 2007.

3. Possley, *The Brown's Chicken Massacre*, p. 166.

4. *Chicago Tribune*, April 13, 2007.

5. Henry C. Lee, Timothy Palmbach, and Marilyn Miller, *Henry Lee's Crime Scene Handbook* (San Diego, CA: Academic Press, 2001), pp. 19, 25.

6. *Chicago Tribune*, April 2, 2007.

7. Dr. Henry Lee, Report, Forensic Research Training Center, Branford, CT, February 8, 2007.

8. Press release, Better Government Association, April 17, 1996.

9. Ibid.

10. Ibid.

11. *Police Chief Magazine*, p. 2.

12. Possley, *The Brown's Chicken Massacre*, p. 130.

13. Ibid., p. 132.

14. Ibid., p. 155.

15. Ibid., p. 201.

16. Ibid., p. 202.

17. Ibid., p. 203.

18. Ibid., p. 205.

19. Ibid., p. 219.

20. Ibid., p. 221.

21. Ibid., p. 224.

22. Ibid., p. 225.

23. Ibid., p. 228.

24. *Chicago Tribune*, March 27, 2007.

25. Ibid.

26. Ibid.

27. Ibid.

28. Possley, *The Brown's Chicken Massacre*, p. 236.

29. Ibid., p. 237.

30. Ibid., pp. 237–38.

31. Ibid., p. 240.

32. NBC Chicago, NBC5.com, May 21, 2002.

33. Ibid.

34. Possley, *The Brown's Chicken Massacre*, p. 242.

35. Ibid., p. 243.

36. NBC Chicago, NBC5.com, May 17, 2002.

37. Possley, *The Brown's Chicken Massacre*, p. 242.

38. Ibid.

39. Ibid., p. 243.

40. PalatineNews5, June 11, 2002.

41. NBC Chicago, NBC5.com, May 21, 2002.

42. Sean P. Mactire, *Malicious Intent* (Cincinnati, OH: Writer's Digest Books, 1995), p. 26.

43. NBC Chicago, NBC5.com, May 19, 2002.

44. Possley, *The Brown's Chicken Massacre*, p. 254.

45. Ibid., p. 255.

46. CBS, March 27, 2007.

47. Ibid.

48. CBS, April 13, 2007.

49. Ibid.

50. *Chicago Tribune*, April 17, 2007.

51. Ibid.

52. *Chicago Sun-Times*, April 19, 2007.

53. *Chicago Tribune*, April 19, 2007.

54. Ibid.

55. *Chicago Tribune*, April 20, 2007.

56. Ibid.

57. *Chicago Tribune*, April 24, 2007.

58. Ibid.

59. *Daily Herald*, April 30, 2007.

60. CBS, May 9, 2007.

61. Ibid.

62. CBS, May 10, 2007.

63. CBS, May 9, 2007.

CHAPTER 3: MURDER IN THE SACRISTY

1. John Glatt, *Forgive Me, Father* (New York: St. Martin's, 2008), p. 45.

2. Ibid., p. 46.

3. Official report of Detective Arthur Marx, April 5, 1980.

4. Ibid.

5. *Toledo Blade*, April 5, 1980.

6. Glatt, *Forgive Me, Father*, p. 65.

7. Ibid., p. 77.

8. Ibid., pp. 104–105.

9. Ibid., pp. 113–14.

10. Fred Rosen, *When Satan Wore a Cross* (New York: HarperCollins, 2007), p. 90.

11. Ibid., p. 97.

12. Glatt, *Forgive Me, Father*, p. 131.

13. Rosen, *When Satan Wore a Cross*, p. 183.

14. Glatt, *Forgive Me, Father*, pp. 133–34.

15. Ibid., pp. 130–31.

16. Rosen, *When Satan Wore a Cross*, pp. 111–12.

17. Glatt, *Forgive Me, Father*, p. 224.

18. Ibid., p. 5.

19. Lucas County Coroner's Office, Autopsy Report on Sister Margaret Ann Pahl, April 5, 1980.

20. Glatt, *Forgive Me, Father*, p. 77.

21. Ibid., pp. 92–93.

22. Ibid., p. 108.

23. Ibid., pp. 98–99.

24. Ibid., p. 103.

25. Ibid., p. 115.

26. Ibid., p. 116.

27. Ibid., p. 141.

28. Ibid., p. 142.

29. Ibid., p. 175.

30. *Toledo Blade*, April 29, 2004.

31. Glatt, *Forgive Me, Father*, p. 190.

32. Vincent J. M. Di Maio and Suzanna E. Dana, *Forensic Pathology* (Austin, TX: Landes Bioscience, 1998), p. 95.

33. Ibid., pp. 97–100.

34. Glatt, *Forgive Me, Father*, p. 236.

35. CourtTVNews, April 26, 2006.

36. Glatt, *Forgive Me, Father*, p. 241.

37. Ibid., pp. 249–50.

38. Ibid., pp. 251–53.

39. CourtTVNews, April 26, 2006.

40. CourtTVNews, May 2, 2006.

41. Glatt, *Forgive Me, Father*, p. 271.

42. Ibid., pp. 275–76.

43. CourtTVNews, May 10, 2006.

44. Glatt, *Forgive Me, Father*, pp. 281, 286.

45. Ibid., pp. 287–90.

46. WTVG, Toledo, OH, 13abc.com, May 12, 2006.

47. Glatt, *Forgive Me, Father*, p. 174.

CHAPTER 4: A POLICE SHOOTING AND THE PUBLIC TRUST

1. *Hartford Courant*, February 15, 2000.

2. *Journal Inquirer*, June 29, 1999.

3. Ibid.

4. *Hartford Courant*, April 17, 1999.

5. *Hartford Courant*, July 2, 1999.

6. Ibid.

7. Ibid.

8. Ibid.

9. *Hartford Courant*, April 17, 1999.

10. Connecticut State Police, Eastern District Major Crime Squad, Investigative Report, June 15, 1999.

11. Ibid.

12. State of Connecticut, Department of Public Safety, State Police Forensic Science Laboratory, Laboratory Case #ID-99–001213, May 21, 1999.

13. *Hartford Courant,* June 17, 1999.

14. *Hartford Courant,* February 15, 2000.

15. *Mr. District Attorney* radio program, circa 1948, personal recollection.

CHAPTER 5: ATROCITIES IN BOSNIA AND CROATIA

1. Center for Balkan Development/Friends of Bosnia, www.friendsof bosnia.org, April 1999.

2. Information Please Database, 2007.

3. *Newsweek,* April 9, 2001.

4. NPR, March 12, 2002.

5. US State Department, *Ethnic Cleansing in Kosovo: An Accounting,* December 1999.

6. "Case Study: Bosnia-Herzegovina," Gendercide Watch, http://www .gendercide.org/case_bosnia.html.

7. Mark Danner, "Bosnia: The Great Betrayal," *New York Review of Books,* March 1998.

8. http://www.gendercide.org/case-bosnia.html.

9. Roger Cohen, "Ethnic Cleansing," Crimes of War Project, http://www.crimesofwar.org/thebook/ethnic-cleansing.html.

10. Charles Krauthammer, "When Serbs Are 'Cleansed,' Moralists Stay Silent," *International Herald Tribune,* August 12, 1995.

11. Cohen, "Ethnic Cleansing."

12. "New Way to Find Mass Graves in Bosnia," *International Herald Tribune,* August 17, 2005.

13. Ibid.

14. Gendercide Watch, http://www.gendercide.org, 1999–2000.

15. Stephen Talbot, *Srebrenica: The Video of a Wartime Atrocity,* August 13, 2005.

BIBLIOGRAPHY

Andrews, Lori B. *The Clone Age.* New York: Henry Holt, 1999.

Baden, Michael. *Confessions of a Medical Examiner.* New York: Ivy Books, 1989.

Baden, Michael, and Marion Roach. *Dead Reckoning: The New Science of Catching Killers.* New York: Simon & Schuster, 2000.

Bosco, Joseph. *Blood Will Tell.* New York: William Morrow, 1993.

Corvasce, Mauro V., and Joseph R. Paglino. *Modus Operandi.* Cincinnati, OH: Writer's Digest Books, 1995.

DeForest, Peter R., Robert Gaensslen, and Henry C. Lee. *Forensic Science: An Introduction to Criminalistics.* New York: McGraw-Hill, 1983.

Di Maio, Vincent J. M., and Suzanna E. Dana. *Forensic Pathology.* Austin, TX: Landes Bioscience, 1998.

Eckert, William G., and Stuart H. James. *Interpretation of Bloodstain Evidence at Crime Scenes.* New York: Elsevier, 1989.

Erzinclioglu, Zakaria. *Forensics: True Crime Scene Investigations.* New York: Barnes & Noble Books, 2002.

Geberth, Vernon J. *Practical Homicide Investigation.* Boca Raton, FL: CRC Press, 1996.

Giannelli, Paul C., and Edward J. Imwinkelried. *Scientific Evidence.* Charlottesville, VA: Michie, 1993.

Glatt, John. *Forgive Me, Father.* New York: St. Martin's, 2008.

Holmes, Paul. *Retrial: Murder and Dr. Sam Sheppard.* New York: Bantam Books, 1966.

Labriola, Jerry. *Murders at Brent Institute.* Avon, CT: Strong Books, 2003.

————. *The Strange Death of Napoleon Bonaparte.* Avon, CT: Strong Books, 2008.

Lee, Henry C., and Jerry Labriola. *Dr. Henry Lee's Forensic Files.* Amherst, NY: Prometheus Books, 2006.

————. *Famous Crimes Revisited.* Avon, CT: Strong Books, 2001.

Lee, Henry C., Timothy Palmbach, and Marilyn Miller. *Henry Lee's Crime Scene Handbook*. San Diego, CA: Academic Press, 2001.

Mactire, Sean P. *Malicious Intent*. Cincinnati, OH: Writer's Digest Books, 1995.

Newton, Michael. *Armed and Dangerous: A Writer's Guide to Weapons*. Cincinnati, OH: Writer's Digest Books, 1990.

Norris, Joel. *Serial Killers*. London: Arrow Books, 1990.

Possley, Maurice. *The Brown's Chicken Massacre*. New York: Berkley Books, 2003.

Ragle, Larry. *Crime Scene*. New York: Avon Books, 1995.

Rhodes, Richard. *Why They Kill*. New York: Alfred A. Knopf, 1999.

Ridley, Matt. *Genome*. New York: Perennial, 1999.

Rosen, Fred. *When Satan Wore a Cross*. New York: HarperCollins, 2007.

Scranton, Phil, and Kathryn Chadwick. *In the Arms of the Law: Coroners' Inquests and Deaths in Custody*. London: Pluto, 1987.

Wecht, Cyril, and Greg Saitz. *Mortal Evidence*. Amherst, NY: Prometheus Books, 2003.

INDEX